Praise for *50 Simple Ways to Live a Longer Life*

"It all seems so easy, doesn't it? Live well. Live simply. And live longer. Well it is simple and there's science to prove it. Suzanne Bohan and Glenn Thompson outline fifty easy ways to make your life better and back each one up with a credible source. I kept turning every page and you will too."
—Nancy L. Snyderman, MD, Associate Clinical Professor Otolaryngology, University of Pennsylvania, Founder of LLuminari Inc.

"Many health writers will wish they had authored this treasure. The 50 nuggets it offers will both empower and inspire readers to base their decisions about long term health on sound science."
—Barbara Rolls, PhD, professor of nutritional science, Pennsylvania State University and author of *The Volumetrics Eating Plan*

"All persons interested in preventing health problems could benefit from this eminently readable, practical, and scientifically sound book. Health professionals could also gain much from this book, in part by learning ways to explain things in simple language. The authors have ingeniously come up with the impressive number of 50 easily understood pathways to improved health. Many are not only healthful but also pleasurable and likely to enhance enjoyment as well as length of life."
—Arthur Klatsky, MD, cardiologist and research scientist, The Kaiser Permanente Medical Care Program

"Most will find this quick 'journal' so remarkably easy to read as to not put it down until they are done. The scientific data has been reduced to simple chapters with easy-to-understand examples of action that the reader can take to improve their health. There is a lot of practical information, with enough good references that even physicians could use sections of it to give advice and help their patients manage their own health. The web links to more information are generally all well respected, up to date, and scientifically credible sites."
—Allan D. Siefkin, MD, Chief Medical Officer, University of California at Davis Health System Chair, Council on Scientific Affairs, California Medical Association

"*50 Simple Ways to Live a Longer Life* serves as a guide to a healthy life. It is very complete with detailed discussions of important issues. Yet it is written in an easy-to-understand fashion. It covers many important lifestyle issues, as well as common illnesses. This book serves as a guide for a longer, healthier and more enjoyable life. Every home should have this book."
—Samuel Meyers, MD, clinical professor of medicine, Mt. Sinai School of Medicine

"This book is a must read for anyone interested in their own health and the health of their family. It provides 50 simple, easy-to-read recipes for how to prevent serious chronic and deadly diseases from heart disease, diabetes and obesity to common cancers. It is a cookbook for good health."
—Michael F. Holick, PhD, MD; Professor of Medicine, Physiology, and Biophysics; Director, General Clinical Research Center, Boston University Medical Center and author of The UV Advantage

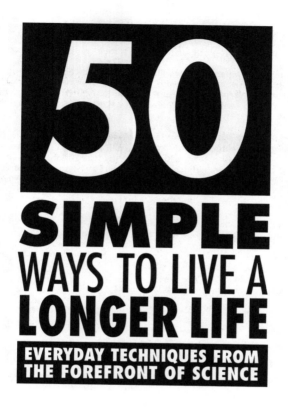

50 SIMPLE
WAYS TO LIVE A
LONGER LIFE

**EVERYDAY TECHNIQUES FROM
THE FOREFRONT OF SCIENCE**

SUZANNE BOHAN
GLENN THOMPSON

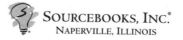

SOURCEBOOKS, INC.®
NAPERVILLE, ILLINOIS

Published by Sourcebooks, Inc.
P.O. Box 4410, Naperville, Illinois 60567-4410
(630) 961-3900
Fax: (630) 961-2168
www.sourcebooks.com

Library of Congress Cataloging-in-Publication Data

Bohan, Suzanne.
  50 simple ways to live a longer life : everyday techniques from the forefront of science / Suzanne Bohan, Glenn Thompson.
       p. cm.
  Includes bibliographical references and index.
  ISBN 1-4022-0375-6 (alk. paper)
  1. Longevity--Popular works. 2. Self-care, Health--Popular works. 3. Aging--Prevention--Popular works. 4. Middle-aged persons--Health and hygiene--Popular works. I. Title: Fifty simple ways to live a longer life. II. Thompson, Glenn. III. Title.

  RA776.75.B64 2005
  612.6'8--dc22

  2005007225

Printed and bound in the United States of America
VP   10   9   8   7   6   5   4   3   2   1

To my mother, Mary Elizabeth Thompson, who taught me to question conventional medical wisdom.
—G. T.

To Grandma Bohan and Uncle Art, who are both still very active in their nineties. Though they may not realize it, they provide a precious link to another time and inspiration to the younger generations in their families.
—S. B.

Contents

Acknowledgments

We wish to thank Ted Weinstein of Ted Weinstein Literary Management for his enthusiasm for the concept behind *50 Simple Ways to Live a Longer Life*. His steady and cheerful professionalism was much appreciated as the book took shape from an idea to a proposal to a finished manuscript. We're also deeply indebted to the scores of distinguished researchers who generously gave their time in interviews. Their participation provided insight and dimension to the book that could never have been achieved without them. We acknowledge the following:

Mark Abramson, MD, instructor, Stanford University School of Medicine

David Allen, personal productivity expert and author

Jeffrey Blumberg, PhD, chief, Antioxidants Research Laboratory, USDA Human Nutrition Research Center on Aging, Tufts University

Walter M. Bortz II, MD, clinical associate professor, Stanford Medical School

Michael Brickey, PhD, psychologist and author

Coralie J.P. Brown, researcher, UC Berkeley

Stephanie Brown, PhD, social psychologist, Institute for Social Research, University of Michigan

Peter Carroll, MD, professor of urology, University of California, San Francisco

Robert C. Colligan, PhD, researcher, Mayo Clinic

Diane Feskanich, ScD, assistant professor, Harvard Medical School

Tiffany Field, PhD, director, The Touch Research Institute, University of Miami School of Medicine

Jane Hightower, MD, internist, California Pacific Medical Center

Michael Holick, MD, PhD, professor of medicine, physiology and biophysics, Boston University Medical Center

Robert Hummer, PhD, director, The Population Center, University of Texas at Austin

Art Klatsky, MD, cardiologist, Kaiser Permanente Medical Center

Clete Kushida, MD, PhD, director, Center for Human Sleep Research, Stanford University

Arthur Levin, MPH, director, Center for Medical Consumers

Becca Levy, PhD, social psychologist, Yale University

Susan Love, MD, breast-cancer specialist and founder, Dr. Susan Love Research Foundation

Mark Mattson, PhD, chief, Laboratory of Neurosciences, National Institute of Aging

Samuel Meyers, MD, clinical professor of medicine, Mt. Sinai School of Medicine

Godfrey Oakley, Jr., MD, MPH, a professor of epidemiology, Emory University

Dean Ornish, MD, director, Preventive Medicine Research Institute, University of California, San Francisco

Jeffrey Potteiger, PhD, chair, Department of Physical Education, Miami University

Barbara Rolls, PhD, professor of nutritional science, Pennsylvania State University

Irwin Rosenberg, MD, senior scientist and director, Nutrition and Neurocognition Laboratory, USDA Human Nutrition Research Center on Aging, Tufts University

Robert Sapolsky, PhD, professor of neuroscience, Stanford University

Carolyn Shaffer, author

Joanne Slavin, PhD, RD, professor, University of Minnesota

Gary Small, MD, director, Center on Aging, University of California, Los Angeles

Michael Thun, MD, head of epidemiological research, American Cancer Society

Cathy Tibbetts, certified diabetes educator, American Diabetes Association

Sara Warber, MD, co-director, Complementary and Alternative Medicine Research Center, University of Michigan

John H. Weisburger, MD, PhD, director emeritus, American Health Foundation

Paul K. Whelton, MD, MSc, senior vice president, Health Sciences, Tulane University

Introduction

Almost daily, news of extraordinary and potentially life-prolonging health advances appears in newspapers and magazines and airs on TV and radio. Yet with so little time, how can anyone expect to learn about, much less digest, this stream of information and then act on it effectively? That's the purpose of this book—to help readers make sense of this information overload and learn how they can use it to enjoy a longer, healthier life. We drew upon hundreds of studies from prestigious medical journals and distilled the research into easy-to-read yet authoritative chapters. Each provides practical advice that empowers you to adopt simple, life-extending, scientifically-based habits. Each short chapter includes a succinct overview, followed by a summary of the latest scientific knowledge, specific suggestions for integrating this knowledge into your life, and references for additional resources.

While in-depth scientific data provides the book's foundation, it's the distinguished experts we interviewed that bring it to life. These accomplished researchers contribute insight and perspective, so valuable when dealing with complicated and often contradictory scientific findings.

As an experienced health journalist and a lifelong health aficionado, we're concerned with bringing busy people health news that can change their lives. We wrote this book in order to condense a large body of medical research into readable, enjoyable, and authoritative prose, to better inform you, the reader.

We selected these 50 topics because they represent the most effective ways people can promote their health and extend their lives. We also covered lesser-known but nonetheless powerful measures that are well-documented to improve health, such as getting more vitamin D, choosing healthful dietary fats, and even increasing self-esteem. Woven throughout this book is the theme that your long-term health and longevity rests in your hands—genes play only a minority role in determining most people's life spans.

The book focuses on practical steps for extending your life and preventing life-threatening diseases. Applying just a few will make an appreciable difference. By adopting even one of the 50 measures outlined here, many others will naturally follow. For example, strengthening your legs will not only increase your mobility and balance in later life, but will improve cardiovascular health, lower your risk of diabetes, and help prevent osteoporosis. Or following the advice to enjoy the stress-reducing effects of nature encourages you to walk more often, which itself confers a myriad of health benefits.

Most people realize that good health is their most important asset. And yet time constraints often prevent people from empowering themselves with knowledge invaluable to their well-being—an endeavor ever more critical with today's costly and fragmented health care system. It's our belief that achieving good health doesn't have to be complicated or time-consuming.

Spending just 10 minutes reading one chapter can show you ways to profoundly influence your health, longevity and well-being. And by living a long, active life, you not only increase your enjoyment during your time on this incredible planet, but you serve as an inspiration and guide for the younger generations in your family.

Suzanne Bohan
Glenn Thompson

CHAPTER 1

Envision a Long Life

Swimmer Megan Quann, winner of two gold medals in the 2000 Olympics at age 16, for years has kept to an unusual bedtime ritual before competitions. Quann lies with her eyes closed, imagining every detail of an upcoming race: The sounds of the crowd, the taste of the water, the view of the bottom of the pool. She then starts a stopwatch as she tensely dives into the pool to begin her imaginary competition. She sees and feels every stroke and every turn. At the race's end, Megan opens her eyes and checks her stopwatch. If she's beat her own actual record or a world record, her envisioned event is a success.

The Olympic swimmer is known as the "poster child for visualization." Visualization is a powerful technique for reducing tension and improving athletic performance. Scores of top athletes practice it. Edwin Moses, a two-time Olympic gold medallist and one of the greatest track stars of all time, would spend time meditating and visualizing before a race. Mary Lou Retton, the first American woman to win an Olympic gold medal in gymnastics, would lie in bed envisioning herself landing straight on the balance beam. Golfing great Jack Nicklaus used to "see" every shot before taking a swing.

Visualization's benefits aren't just confined to athletics. In virtually any endeavor, studies show that taking the time to envision desired outcomes bolsters the chances of success. And that includes envisioning your own life far into the future, while you remain healthy, active, and enjoying life.

Can you see yourself at 80, 90, or even 100, still spry, alert, and active with a caring circle of friends and family? That's the first step you need to take to arrive at a grand old age, still enjoying each day.

What Scientists Know

Creative imagery works by forging connections between thoughts, feelings and ultimately actions. Decades of research with athletes show that visualization improves actual performance. Another 2004 study reports that participants who simply visualized pumping heavy weights had a 13 percent increase in arm strength, without lifting a barbell.

Visualization can even mobilize the body's immune system and help control anxiety and blood pressure, according to studies. A major health insurer now offers guided imagery for patients before surgery, after finding a reduction in hospital and drug costs among patients using the technique.

A 2004 study found that visualization and relaxation techniques helped obese women lose weight and keep it off, without dieting. "It's not just wishful thinking," says Dean Ornish, MD, a bestselling author and director of the Preventive Medicine Research Institute. "It's not 'Oh, if I think it's going to be true, it's going to be true.' Rather, it's a way of mobilizing your full resources and intentions.

"If you imagine yourself as a healthy person," he continues, "then you begin to notice the kinds of resources, evidence, and information that's out there than can enable you to actualize that."

He cites as an example the way a hungry person driving down a highway will notice the restaurants near the road, but pay no attention to the gas stations. "But if you're about to run out of gas, it's the opposite," Ornish says.

David Allen, a personal productivity expert and author of *Getting Things Done*, describes the power of positive imagery in this way: "The bottom line is it makes you more conscious, more focused, and more capable of implementing the changes and results you want, whatever they are."

Making It Real

There are two types of imagery, according to Ornish. One is called directed visualization, and is used to direct images from your conscious mind to your subconscious and to your body's senses. The other is receptive visualization, which helps bring to mind information you've buried or ignored.

To engage in directed visualization, Ornish, in his acclaimed book, *Dr. Dean Ornish's Program for Reversing Heart Disease*, suggests getting into a comfortable position, closing your eyes, and using two or more of your senses—sight, sound, touch, smell and taste. Some ideas for directly envisioning a long, happy life includes imagining the way you'll look and sound when you're older, the activities you'll participate in, the hugs of friends and family in the future, or the taste of your favorite drink as you relax, watch a sunset, and reflect on your long, successful life. Then add more detail, to include images of a healthy heart, sharp, alert mind, strong muscles, and a ready smile.

When you're done visualizing, you may feel profoundly affected, and consider the things you can do now to start achieving those visions—building good relationships with friends and family, strength training regularly, eating more fruits and vegetables, losing a few pounds. The list is endless.

To perform receptive visualization, pose questions to yourself, such as, "What steps can I take to preserve and enhance my health in the coming decades?" Receptive imagery can "help you access information we all carry around with us which tends to speak very clearly but quietly, but often gets drowned out in the chatter of every-day life," Ornish explains.

In the following 49 chapters, you'll find scores of proven ways to help you live a longer, happier life. Envision doing them now.

TO LEARN MORE

In the book *Dr. Dean Ornish's Program for Reversing Heart Disease*, read the chapter entitled "Opening Your Heart to Feelings and to Inner Peace."

Also visit the website of Health Journeys, a group that develops guided imagery tools, at www.healthjourneys.com. Type in either "visualization" or "guided imagery" in the search box.

CHAPTER 2

Stay Hungry

One of the most remarkable recommendations in this book is this: Stay hungry more often, and you may just outlive your peers. And, as a bonus, you'll feel more energetic along the way while you may delay signs of aging like wrinkled skin, hair loss, heart disease, and mental decline.

If that sounds too good to be true, consider the findings from decades of animal research, from rodents to our close cousins, the primates.

In 1935, a Cornell University scientist named Clive McCay first called attention to the link between a modest diet and longevity when he showed that rodents fed a low-calorie, nutrient-rich diet dramatically outlived normally fed rats. Even after the last rat on the normal eating plan died, most of the rats on the restricted diet were still vigorous, alert and sexually active. The oldest rats in this group survived to 1,800 days, the equivalent of 150 human years.

Since then, scientists have conducted more than 2,000 diet restriction animal studies. The research consistently shows that animals on a restricted diet have far longer life spans than their food-satiated counterparts. As a rule, a 30 percent reduction in caloric intake corresponded to at least a 30 percent increase in life span in these studies.

These dramatic findings prompted the prestigious National Institutes of Health to begin a costly diet restriction study on primates. Thus far, the results are encouraging. The primates on the calorie-reduced diet appear healthier, more alert, and seem to be outliving their fully fed peers, according to Mark Mattson, PhD, an NIH scientist.

And a population of long-lived, robust Japanese supports the theory that restricting food intake will also slow the aging process in humans. Residents of the island of Okinawa boast over three times the number of centenarians as their counterparts on the Japanese mainland.

The Okinawans, it was found, consume about one-third fewer calories than other Japanese. Not only do they live longer on average, Okinawans also have significantly lower rates of cancer, heart disease, diabetes, high blood pressure, and cognitive decline, compared with other Japanese.

What Scientists Know

The late Roy Walford, MD, a University of California, Los Angeles scientist who was a leading authority on calorie restriction, began studying the link between calorie restriction and longevity in the 1970s. Walford, who wrote several other books and countless scholarly articles, explains the phenomenon in his 2000 book, *Beyond the 120 Year Diet.* The most widely accepted hypothesis explaining the longevity effect of calorie restriction involves free radicals or unstable molecules, which studies show damage cellular membranes and DNA. By eating less, fewer free radicals (a natural by-product of metabolism) are produced and less damage is done. It's this damage over time that contributes to the aging process.

Another explanation holds that as we eat less, we lower our levels of blood glucose (sugar). While glucose fuels our body's cells, excess amounts slowly "gum up" cellular proteins and bog down the system. Indeed, it's these blood sugar-protein interactions that cause diabetics their health problems such as heart disease and cataracts.

A third hypothesis holds that calorie restriction stresses the body's cells. This leads to an adaptation which strengthens the body against future environmental assaults and ultimately slows metabolism and the aging process.

Making It Real

In his book, Walford describes a low-calorie eating plan that lops off a third of the calories from a typical diet. The advice is familiar: Consume generous servings of vegetables and fruits, eat 40 to 80 grams of lean protein a day, and select nutritionally dense foods like whole grain breads, brown rice, buckwheat, nuts, and legumes.

He warns that his plan is not for the faint of heart, but claims that the rewards are immense, including a renewed feeling of vitality, the slowing of the aging process, and the postponement or prevention of chronic diseases.

But because such a drastic cut in calories can shock the body and makes achieving a balanced diet all the more difficult, readers are advised to study Walford's plan carefully before proceeding with his or any similar program.

To Learn More

Read the book *Beyond the 120 Year Diet: How to Double Your Vital Years* by Roy Walford, MD.

CHAPTER 3

Skip a Meal

If, as we described in the previous chapter, the idea of carving out a third of your daily calories holds little appeal, check out these new findings on "meal skipping."

Mark Mattson, PhD, a scientist with the National Institute on Aging (a division of the National Institutes of Health), tested the effect of food restriction and health on three groups of rodents: those that were permitted to eat freely; those on a calorie-restricted plan in which they ate 30 percent less than the free-eating group; and a third group of "intermittent-fasting" rodents that were given all the food they wanted one day, and then none the next.

In a recent journal article, Mattson describes the results. While no one was surprised that the calorie-restricted mice outlived their free-eating peers, the remarkable finding was that the "fasting" rodents fared even slightly better than the calorie-restricted mice. Both lived a third longer than the mice that ate as they pleased. But the fasting rodents actually had lower blood levels of glucose and insulin than the calorie-restricted mice. An excess of either of these compounds is associated with diseases like heart disease and diabetes.

And it wasn't because the fasting mice became thinner. While the calorie-restricted mice lost 30 percent of their weight, the fasting mice didn't lose any, since they ate twice as much as food on the days they could eat freely.

In a 2003 study with lab animals, Mattson found that intermittent fasting was as effective as regular exercise in reducing blood pressure, heart rate, and insulin levels.

What Scientists Know

The body's cells are like muscles, says Mattson. Both are strengthened by a little stress.

"If you stress your muscles by exercising them, they become stronger and more resistant to injury," he says. "This is essentially what's going on with cells throughout the body by intermittent fasting."

This "nutritional stress" causes cells to change their metabolism, Mattson explains. The stress of a brief fast generates proteins which protect and strengthen the body against stress.

Studies show direct evidence that both calorie restriction and eating fewer than three meals a day "primes the cells to handle more severe kinds of stress."

Scientists aren't yet certain how nutritional stress delays the aging process. However, Mattson says there's evidence that rates of cell division and cell death are slowed down with dietary restriction. He also says studies show that cells that don't divide, such as brain cells, become resistant to degeneration during aging in animals regularly following intermittent fasts.

Making It Real

No one is advising that people adopt an every-other-day fasting regimen. Few could sustain it, and fasting often leads to irritability and fatigue. While his research findings are bound to stir debate among nutritionists, Mattson says that scaling back to two meals, or even one meal, per day may offer a proportional benefit to an all-day fast. And he advises adopting the diet gradually.

"If you can wean yourself onto it over a couple of months, your body adjusts to it," Mattson says. "Once you're adapted to it, not only will it not be detrimental, it will be beneficial."

Mattson also warns that only those currently in good health should embark on this new eating approach. People living with chronic ailments like diabetes, heart disease, or AIDS should always talk with their doctor before making any significant changes in their diet.

Mattson's own day goes like this: He works out in the morning, but doesn't eat breakfast (and hasn't for 20 years). He then eats a light lunch and a full dinner. At 5' 9", Mattson weighs 125 pounds and has a body mass index of 18. He says he never feels weak in the morning, and emphasizes that the body gets used to such an eating style. In fact, throughout most of history, many humans ate similarly, according to Mattson.

"The diet we currently eat is very abnormal if you look at our evolutionary history. We didn't always eat exactly three meals a day all the time," he says. "Our systems are geared to go without food for much more than six to eight hours. It's not a big deal."

Expect to hear more about the impact of meal skipping and human health, as Mattson and his colleagues at the NIA and USDA have launched a human study on intermittent fasting.

To Learn More

Visit the National Institute of Aging's website at www.nia.nih.gov and type "intermittent fasting" in the search box.

CHAPTER 4

Walk Through a Long Life

Throughout history, people have instinctively recognized the salutary effects of the simple activity of walking. As the ancient Greek physician Hippocrates put it so succinctly, "Walking is man's best medicine."

Over the last few decades, scientists have confirmed just how right he was. The more we learn about walking, the more remarkable this easy, pleasurable activity becomes. Long disregarded as a bona fide form of exercise, it's emerging as one of the most esteemed ways to stay fit.

Walking offers immediate pleasures, as you can enjoy the out-of-doors, new sights, and time to think or to visit with a companion. And when you're finished, you'll invariably feel better, physically and mentally.

That's welcome news for the legions of harried people who know they need to fit more exercise into their lives, but find it difficult to go to a gym. Instead, walkers can easily integrate the activity into their daily lives, while also enjoying the tranquility and physical health it delivers.

What Scientists Know

A regular walking routine will protect you from a range of debilitating conditions.

Harvard Medical School researchers studied the lifestyle patterns of more than 70,000 women and found that even 30 minutes a day of brisk walking reduced a woman's heart attack risk by as much as 40 percent. Make that 45 minutes a day, and the risk of heart attack drops by half.

Walking has also proven itself equal to vigorous exercise. The risk reduction for heart attacks was the same for women who walked three hours per week and those who spent one-and-a-half hours every week engaged in more vigorous activities like biking, running or swimming. In an encouraging finding for lifelong couch potatoes, the researchers also found that previously sedentary adults who embarked on a walking routine dramatically improved their health.

Another Harvard study of 11,000 men reports that those who briskly walked 30 minutes a day, five days a week, cut their stroke risk by a quarter. Those that doubled that walking rate cut their odds by half. A 2004 study found that walking two or three days a week improved blood flow to the brain, resulting in improved memory, learning ability, and attentiveness. Another study of 60,000 women links regular walking with stronger leg bones and lower rates of osteoporotic fractures.

And the benefits of walking don't end there. A federal government report called "Stepping Out" notes that walking also reduces the risk of developing diabetes, high blood pressure, and colon and breast cancers; helps to maintain normal weight, as well as healthy bones, muscles, and joints; increases production of growth hormones that counteract the effects of aging; strengthens reflexes, making you less prone to debilitating accidents like falling; and increases the production of endorphins, which reduce feelings of depression and anxiety, while promoting a sense of well-being.

Making It Real

Early American educator Horace Mann wrote, "Habit is a cable; we weave a thread of it each day, and at last we cannot break it." To develop this healthy habit, just try walking every day, even for a few minutes. You'll likely soon start looking forward to getting outside for a break. And keep a brisk pace; one study showed leisurely strollers didn't gain much in health benefits.

Always start off easy and build up, increasing your activity level about 20 percent each week until you arrive at your desired level. If you join or start a walking club, you'll find extra support and maybe make some new friendships over the miles.

The good news is that if you can't squeeze long walks into your schedule, research shows that short bouts of exercise are as effective as regular workouts in all regards except for achieving weight loss. (For that, you need regular sustained workouts.)

The opportunities are endless. Get off the bus one stop early, walk for 15 minutes at lunchtime, walk around the airport while waiting for a plane or do a lap while at your child's soccer game. Take the stairs whenever possible. To add an extra dimension to your workout, carry light dumbbells to strengthen arm muscles.

Keep an alternate place in mind to walk during inclement weather, like an indoor shopping mall. You can also integrate walking into volunteer activities; try acting as a museum or hiking docent.

To Learn More

Visit the President's Council on Physical Fitness and Sports' information-packed website at www.fitness.gov.

The National Highway Traffic Safety Administration has a terrific guide, called "Stepping Out," on the health benefits of walking. The report is interspersed with advice for keeping safe while walking. Find it at www.nhtsa.dot.gov/people/injury/olddrive/SteppingOut.

CHAPTER 5

Defy the Stereotypes

By refusing to accept the ubiquitous and negative stereotypes about aging, you'll almost certainly live a happier life. That act of defiance may also keep you around longer to enjoy those more fulfilling days. Positive words and expectations have a profound effect on the health, memory, mobility and even life span of elders, according to a slew of recent findings. But maintaining upbeat expectations about your golden years can be hard to achieve in youth-obsessed, elder-denigrating America.

"The stereotype is it's all downhill and life gets worse," says Michael Brickey, PhD, the author of *Defy Aging* and a popular speaker about living a long, vibrant life. "The data seems to suggest the opposite, that older people report being happy," he adds. "With age, we tend to get more wisdom and we place more value on friendships."

The irony of this dim view of aging is that, if we're lucky, we'll all live to an old age. Yet waiting to haunt us will be our own negative views about growing old. If a mix of compassion and enlightened self interest isn't enough to shift American society toward a more holistic outlook on the aging process, then perhaps the realization that it could save big bucks in health care spending will.

A number of studies strongly suggest that chronic stress in older Americans is caused in part by negative stereotypes. Chronic stress is linked to health problems such as high blood pressure, heart disease, and dementia, which add billions of dollars per year to the nation's health care bill. Another study suggests that oppressed elders are also more likely to have poor balance and suffer costly and debilitating fractures.

What Scientists Know

"Friendly," "funny," and "kind." These were the words used most often by a group of young Chinese adults when describing a group of elder Chinese. In China, dictums dating from the time of Confucius instruct that elders be treated with respect and reverence.

"Decrepit," "cranky," and "wrinkled." Those were the words used by a group of young American adults when describing a group of older Americans, where negative views of the elderly abound in popular culture.

And guess what happened when the older adults had their memory tested against the younger members of their ethnic group? The elder Chinese scored as well as the younger Chinese, while the elder Americans scored much worse than their younger counterparts. Another test on Americans confirmed that positive messages about aging improved memory in older people. "People of all ages are forgetful," emphasizes Becca Levy, PhD, a social psychologist at Yale University who conducted both memory studies.

"What most people call 'senior moments' is really stress," notes Brickey. "Anybody experiencing a lot of stress is going to have difficulty with recall at any age."

In a test of the physical effect on elders of positive words like "wise" and "astute" and negative words like "senile" or "diseased," researchers found that those subliminally viewing the uplifting words walked significantly faster than those flashed discouraging words. Why is walking fast important? The study notes that as older people slow down their pace, their balance isn't as sure and they're more likely to fall, increasing their risk of suffering a debilitating fracture.

Optimistic expectations about aging even increase life spans. A long-term study of Ohio residents found that those who disagreed with statements like, "as you get older, you are less useful," lived on average 7.5 years longer than those who accepted that negative stereotype. That's a bigger gain in longevity than you'd get by taking blood pressure- or cholesterol-lowering drugs.

In other research, the blood pressure climbed in older people hearing negative stereotypes about aging, while dropping in those getting positive messages.

Making It Real

Defying age-related stereotypes isn't for the faint of heart.

"It's a challenge to overcome," Levy says. "But it's possible."

The socially sanctioned degradation of the elderly "becomes most obvious when you look at humor," says Brickey. "A high percentage of humor about older people is very negative, and people tend to believe it." He advises ignoring such negative jokes. "Just regard them as garbage and reject them out of hand," he says. "I pounce right on people when they talk about 'senior moments,'" Brickey adds. "It's very destructive."

He counters that stereotype by comparing the mind to a computer, which becomes richer and fuller with age. "So what if your megahertz is a little slower? Would you really want to trade that for a scrawny hard drive with a little bit of information and a few programs on it?" Brickey counsels people to tell themselves a phrase like "it will come to me" if they can't recall something, and that often it soon does. He advises using the power of the pen to fight back against age-related stereotypes. After hearing an offensive remark, he suggests writing down a list of retorts you wish you had said. (The French call that "staircase wit," those responses that come to mind only as you're leaving down the stairs.)

"These remarks tend to be repetitive, so you have your retort handy and you just zing them with it, the way that Ronald Reagan did in the debates," Brickey says. During the 1984 presidential debate with Walter Mondale, Reagan quipped in response to concerns about his age that, "I will not make age an issue of this campaign. I am not going to exploit, for political purposes, my opponent's youth and inexperience."

"He had his comeback ready, and it worked brilliantly," Brickey says.

To Learn More

Read the American Psychological Association's "Resolution on Aging" on its website at www.apa.org/pi/aging/ageism.html. On the page, click on "Publications" to find additional reading on the topic.

Read Michael Brickey's *Defy Aging*. Visit his website at www.drbrickey.com to sign up for a free subscription to the Defy Aging Newsletter.

CHAPTER 6

Supplement Smartly

Few examples better illustrate mainstream medicine's historical aversion toward vitamin supplementation than the story of the slow acceptance of life-saving folic acid. As early as the end of World War II, scientists were linking folic acid deficiency with devastating central nervous system deformities in fetuses, particularly spina bifida. But 50 years would pass, and countless deformed infants would be born, before doctors began routinely advising women of childbearing age to supplement with folic acid.

The tide is turning, as underscored in a 2002 report in the *Journal of the American Medical Association* that concluded that all adults should take a daily multivitamin to help prevent chronic diseases. But word is spreading slowly among health experts, many of whom still believe that a balanced diet provides all the nutrients you need.

That's "patently ridiculous," says Jeffrey Blumberg, PhD, professor of nutrition at Tufts University and a nationally recognized expert on nutrition and vitamins.

Blumberg, who takes vitamin C, vitamin E, and calcium, says that evidence is "compelling" that vitamin supplements improve health and prevent disease. He adds that "the risks are essentially nil, and the benefits are clear."

What Scientists Know

The *JAMA* report reviewed more than 100 studies and concluded that "most people do not consume an optimal amount of all vitamins by diet alone ... it appears prudent for all adults to take vitamin supplements."

There's little dispute that a balanced diet will prevent the onset of maladies caused by vitamin deficiencies, such as scurvy, beriberi, or rickets. Still, research shows that vitamin intake at "optimal" levels is essential for promoting health and preventing degenerative conditions such as heart disease, stroke, cancer and even cognitive decline. (Optimal levels are higher than the government's Recommended Daily Allowance, or RDAs.)

Famed cancer researcher Bruce Ames, PhD, at the University of California, Berkeley, goes even further. "A deficiency of any of the vitamins—folic acid, vitamin B12, vitamin B6, niacin, vitamin C, vitamin E—cause DNA and chromosomal damage in much the same way as radiation or carcinogenic chemicals," he writes in a 2001 study. This deficiency, he concludes, explains why people with diets low in fruits and vegetables have double the cancer rate of their better-nourished counterparts.

He goes on to note that "remedying these deficiencies, which can be done at low cost, is likely to lead to a major improvement in health and an increase in longevity."

Low levels of folic acid, vitamin B6, or vitamin B12 are risk factors for cardiovascular disease, birth defects, and cancers of the colon and breast; low levels of vitamin D contribute to osteoporosis, breast cancer, and prostate cancer. Low levels of the antioxidant vitamins A, C, and E may increase risk for chronic diseases like heart disease, some cancers and macular degeneration.

Although the debate over supplementing with a well-balanced multivitamin is fading, the practice of "megadosing" with vitamins C and E, and B-vitamins still draws fire, despite compelling evidence of their disease-preventing benefits.

Making It Real

For those interested in moving beyond a multiple vitamin, we've highlighted the research about the typical megadosed vitamins.

Vitamin C, the most publicized, researched, and hyped supplement, has many functions. A well-balanced diet provides sufficient levels to "get along," but achieving optimal levels takes supplementation. Studies suggest that optimal supplementation with vitamin C helps to prevent heart disease, high blood pressure, stroke, some types of cancer and even cataracts. Although daily doses of two to three grams of vitamin C appears well-tolerated and is frequently the starting point for megadosers, that quantity doesn't seem necessary. The Physicians Desk Reference for Supplements concludes that levels of 200 mg/day (four to five times the RDA) is about all your body can use at any one time. Amounts above that are excreted.

Vitamin E, a supplement superstar, has been controversial since its discovery in 1922. It wasn't universally considered an essential nutrient until 1966, and its RDA wasn't established by the federal government until 1968.

Vitamin E is a powerful antioxidant found in egg yolks, some oils, whole grains, and fish. Research shows that supplementing with vitamin E lowers the risk of developing cardiovascular disease, particularly when taken regularly. There's also strong evidence that vitamin E contributes to the prevention of cancers of the prostate and lung. While vitamin E can be taken at levels approaching 1,500 IUs with little or no side effects, that's unnecessary, as most of the preventative benefits peak at 400 IUs per day. Two recent studies have cast doubt on the safety of vitamin E, including a March 2005 study describing potentially adverse effects on cardiovascular health. But Blumberg describes those studies as "deeply flawed" and says that there should be no concern over its safety when taken at recommended dosages.

Vitamin E, vitamin C, and the mineral selenium work synergistically, in which each supplement's benefit is magnified when taken in combination. One warning about vitamin E: it thins the blood and shouldn't be taken with anti-coagulant medications or before surgery without informing your doctor. In addition, anyone taking medications should always talk with a physician about potential interactions between supplements and their prescribed drugs.

Folic acid and vitamin D play such powerful roles in preventing numerous diseases that each has its own chapter: 25 and 24, respectively.

In summary, everyone should take a daily multivitamin, and those interested in bolstering their levels of key nutrients can add 200 mg to 300 mg of vitamin C, 400 IUs of vitamin E, 800 IUs of folic acid, and 800 IUs of vitamin D. Take your vitamins with food to promote absorption and avoid indigestion.

To Learn More

Visit the National Institutes of Health's website on vitamins and minerals at www.nlm.nih.gov/medlineplus/vitaminsandminerals.html. The site offers comprehensive information on supplements, along with new research.

CHAPTER 7

Rediscover Aspirin

Aspirin, humanity's most widely used drug, comes right from nature's medicine chest.

The active ingredient in aspirin, acetylsalicylic acid, was originally derived from plants like willow, birch, and myrtle. Plants use the compound to protect against pathogens; in humans, it's long been used to ease minor discomforts.

Around 3000 BC, ancient Egyptian physicians brewed willow tea to treat aches and pains. Greek and Roman healers, from Hippocrates to Galen, carried on that tradition. Native Americans used birch to ease toothaches. Modern aspirin was invented in 1897 by Felix Hoffman, a chemist for Bayer AG who was seeking a remedy for his father's painful rheumatoid arthritis.

Among the first reports of aspirin's greater potential came in the 1950s, when a California doctor published a study showing that it protected heart attack patients from a second attack. The work appeared in an obscure journal and received little notice. But the world paid attention when a prominent British heart specialist in 1974 reported that heart attack patients taking a daily dose of aspirin cut their risk of a second heart attack by one fourth.

Since 1974, numerous studies have confirmed aspirin's striking effectiveness in protecting people from cardiovascular disease. Each day, 80 million aspirin are taken in the United States, with at least half of those consumed for heart attack and stroke prevention.

But the amazing health-promoting qualities of this inexpensive white pill don't seem to quit. Aspirin, the "wonder drug" of the 20th century, is poised to reclaim the title in the 21st century, according to many experts. Aspirin has been linked to lowered risk of developing numerous types of cancer: a 28 percent drop in breast cancer risk; up to a 50 percent reduction in the risk of developing colon cancer; a 20 percent drop for ovarian cancer; and roughly fifty percent declines for leukemia, melanoma and cancers of the stomach and esophagus. Preliminary evidence suggests that aspirin also plays a role in preventing bladder cancer, and may thwart the development of Alzheimer's disease. In a new therapeutic twist, a 2003 study from Dartmouth University reported that aspirin reduced rates of staph infections, an increasing threat in hospitals.

What Scientists Know

Much of aspirin's seemingly miraculous work comes from its ability to block the production of prostaglandins, hormone-like substances essential to causing sensations of pain. Prostaglandins also promote blood flow to injured or infected areas, hence causing the uncomfortable swelling associated with inflammation. By inhibiting prostaglandin production, aspirin blocks both sensations of pain and the development of sore, inflamed areas. Aspirin's heart-protective effect arises from its ability to stop blood platelets from sticking together. That thins the blood and keeps it flowing through arteries partially blocked by plaque buildup, reducing incidents of heart attack and stroke. It's also believed to ease inflammation of artery walls, which triggers the buildup of deadly plaque.

Researchers aren't certain yet how aspirin might prevent cancer, but the area is under intense study. Prostaglandins promote estrogen production, and increased estrogen levels are directly linked to breast cancer risk. So, aspirin's well-known activity in blocking prostaglandin formation may also serve to protect against breast cancer. With other kinds of cancer, like those of the colon and prostate, new evidence suggests that aspirin activates the body's immune system, inhibiting the spread of cancer cells.

Scientists think aspirin's anti-inflammatory activity could explain its potential preventive effect against Alzheimer's disease. It may also block brain enzymes thought to promote the buildup of amyloid plaque, damaging deposits that accumulate in the brain cells of people with Alzheimer's disease.

Making It Real

Since the 1980s, the FDA has recommended aspirin for preventing a subsequent heart attack or stroke in those who've already had one. In 2002, the federal government expanded its guidelines to recommend regular consumption of low dose aspirin for those who haven't had a heart attack, but are at higher than average risk of developing one.

Because studies on aspirin's cancer protective effects are still considered preliminary, and aspirin is not risk-free, no major health organization is ready to recommend its use for cancer prevention. In a very small percentage of people, aspirin may lead to gastrointestinal bleeding or hemorrhagic stroke.

But most health experts also recognize that, with aspirin's promising role in protecting against certain cancers, people will decide to self-treat. The FDA even requires drug makers to note on aspirin labels that "serious side effects could occur with self treatment."

"Certainly people can make their own decisions," says Michael Thun, MD, the head of epidemiological research for the American Cancer Society. "But it's quite another thing for health organizations to make decisions based on (scientific) evidence.

"People in general don't think of baby aspirin or aspirin the way they do other drugs," he continues. "So they may not take seriously the fact that there can be serious side effects."

And there are many people who shouldn't take aspirin, or should do so cautiously, because of chronic diseases such as asthma or lifestyle reasons like heavy drinking. Pregnant women should not take aspirin.

Bottom line: If you're thinking about taking aspirin every day, for the rest of your life, don't make that decision lightly. It's a potent medicine. Always talk with your doctor about its risks and benefits, given your age and medical profile.

To Learn More

Visit the FDA's online "Questions and Answers" page about aspirin at www.fda.gov/cder/news/aspirin/aspirin_qa.htm.

CHAPTER 8

Build Strong Bones

Most Americans are too complacent about their odds of developing osteoporosis, a debilitating disease that so weakens the bones that just swinging a golf club or doing heavy chores could fracture a vertebrae, wrist or hip. A 2004 Roper survey found that only 15 percent of women with risk factors for osteoporosis consider themselves vulnerable to the bone-wasting condition. And most men aren't much better, dubbing osteoporosis a "women's disease" according to a Gallup Poll.

So what's the reality? A stunning 50 percent of women and 25 percent of men will develop a fracture due to osteoporosis during their lifetime, according to the National Institutes of Health. Few diseases have such reach in the United States. Each year, osteoporosis causes 1.5 million broken bones. Of those, 300,000 are hip fractures, which ultimately kill one quarter of the victims within a year.

Despite widespread advertising claims about calcium consumption and bone health, drinking more milk and swallowing more calcium pills isn't the alpha and the omega of preventing osteoporosis. In fact, research on their effectiveness is decidedly mixed, according to Diane Feskanich, ScD, a researcher with Harvard Medical School who focuses on dietary influences in the development of osteoporosis.

Feskanich points out the paradox revealed by worldwide patterns of osteoporosis. Scandinavian countries have high levels of dairy consumption, but she says they also have the highest rates of osteoporosis. In contrast, in Asian countries, where dairy products are rarely consumed, rates of osteoporosis are among the lowest in the world. "The focus on calcium is overdone," Feskanich says. In fact, the 52-year-old scientist—who, tests show, has strong bone density—doesn't even take calcium supplements. She instead relies on exercise and adequate vitamin D intake to counter the slow bone loss that begins in adults after age 30.

What Scientists Know

A growing number of researchers, including Feskanich, believe that a shortage of vitamin D is one of the real culprits behind osteoporosis. In fact, studies of calcium's role in preventing fractures only showed a reduction when vitamin D was also provided to participants.

Without the "sunshine vitamin," most calcium would pass through the body unused. (See chapter 24 to learn more about the crucial role of vitamin D in disease prevention.) Vitamin D is vital for effective absorption of dietary calcium. Even with vitamin D fortification of dairy products and other foods, vitamin D deficiency is rampant in the United States, writes Michael Holick, MD, PhD, the director of the Vitamin D Research Lab at Boston University Medical Center, in a 2003 study. Admonitions to avoid the sun are one reason for this widespread deficiency. While the advice is largely sound, UV rays trigger the formation of vitamin D, and short periods of exposure (10 to 15 minutes a day for most people) are healthy.

Besides getting enough vitamin D, add exercise to your routine. It's one of the most effective approaches to reducing bone loss, Feskanich says. Despite their rigid appearance, bones are living tissue that need physical stress to remain strong and healthy. That's why astronauts lose significant bone mass while in a zero-gravity environment.

When you run or lift weights, chemical messengers send signals that foster bone growth, enabling the bone to handle greater loads in the future. Studies of professional tennis players show that bones in their playing arms are significantly larger and denser than those in the non-playing arms. A physically vigorous lifestyle even proved as effective as now-controversial hormone replacement therapy in protecting women against osteoporosis, Feskanich emphasizes.

Another cause of osteoporosis is low intake of vitamin K, which is found in most leafy green vegetables. Vitamin K performs a key role in the formation of bone protein, and deficiencies are linked to significantly higher rates of hip fractures.

Excess protein consumption is associated with osteoporosis, as it creates an acidic environment that draws calcium from bone. But don't cut back too much, as moderate levels of protein promote bone health. Elevated levels of homocysteine, a by-product of meat digestion, are also newly linked with high hip fracture rates. While there's excitement about the potential benefits of soy and bone health, Feskanich says research is inconclusive on that issue. Nor is moderate consumption of coffee and soda convincingly linked to bone deterioration.

Making It Real

Exercise is the premier osteoporosis prevention strategy, Feskanich emphasizes. She's worked out daily for 30 years, and has strong bones as a result, she's certain. "Exercise, at all ages, is the best thing," she says.

Feskanich isn't a naysayer about dairy foods—she just thinks their benefit in preventing osteoporosis has been overblown. "I don't have anything against dairy products," she says. "But I wouldn't tell people they have to have them." She eats yogurt regularly to make sure she gets enough calcium, but says consuming supplements or foods supplemented with calcium can also provide adequate amounts.

Milk is also fortified with retinol, the animal-based form of vitamin A. One explanation for the high prevalence of osteoporosis in Scandanavian countries, despite the high consumption of dairy products there, may be the vitamin A fortification of milk, Feskanich says. While moderate amounts of vitamin A are essential for good bone health, studies also strongly link excess vitamin A consumption with an increased rate of hip fracture. "Milk is kind of a mixed bag for that reason," she explains.

The bottom line on calcium: make sure to get adequate levels, about 1,000 mg a day. In addition to dairy products, green leafy vegetables such as broccoli, collards, kale, mustard greens, turnip greens, and bok choy are good sources of calcium. Salmon and sardines canned with their soft bones are other good sources. But pair calcium intake with adequate vitamin D levels, at least 400 IUs a day, and as much as 800 IUs.

To Learn More

The National Osteoporosis Foundation offers an information-packed website, including links to other sources: www.nof.org.

CHAPTER 9

Stay Connected

In the early 1960s, researchers noticed something remarkable about the town of Roseto, Pennsylvania. People in the small, close-knit Italian-American community had less than one sixth the rate of heart disease than the average American, yet they ate more red meat and fatty foods. They also had about the same levels of high blood pressure, obesity and stress.

After years of study, medical experts narrowed this puzzling scenario to one factor: the citizens of Roseto enjoyed strong family ties, elders were accorded a high degree of respect, and a sense of unconditional support infused the community, according to Stewart Wolf, the director of the study.

But when the younger generation migrated to distant subdivisions, the community cohesion began to unravel. In tandem, rates of heart disease steadily climbed, and by the mid-1970s mirrored those of the rest of the country.

Many other studies show similar findings: Socially isolated people develop more chronic diseases, and succumb more readily to them. The quality of our human relationships even fuels our motivation to achieve health and well being. "Telling somebody who's lonely and depressed that they can live longer if they just change their diet or exercise isn't that motivating," says Dean Ornish, MD, bestselling author and director of the Preventive Medicine Research Institute. "Who wants to live longer if you're not happy?"

What Scientists Know

One of the largest studies on social ties and longevity comes from Alameda County in California, where a study of nearly 7,000 people found that those with the least connections to other people died at two to three times the rate as people with rich social lives.

At Duke University Medical Center, research found that heart disease patients without a spouse or close friend died at three times the rate of those with close emotional support.

An investigation of the entire population of Norway revealed that marriage bestowed a 15 percent survival advantage for people living with cancer. Other studies link social isolation with susceptibility to infectious diseases, arthritis, and epileptic seizures. Strong social ties can even boost immune system function, lower blood pressure, and reduce stress levels.

Some of the health boost from a wide circle of friends and family may arise from simple pragmatic reasons. People with strong social networks have greater access to health information, such as where to go for health care and which doctor to see. They also provide each other with financial assistance and help with matters like transportation to healthcare facilities. People in a bonded primary relationship tend to eat better, and engage in less risky behavior like excessive drinking.

But research also reveals that you need to choose social companions wisely. Spending time with people you don't trust or people who act competitively or rudely can do more harm than good. Utah students who wore concealed monitors exhibited elevated blood pressure levels after interacting with people who aroused negative feelings in them. Scores of other studies show non-supportive social ties lowered immune system function or stressed cardiovascular function as much as social isolation.

Recent research also suggests that it's the quality, not quantity, of your social circle that makes the difference. University of Michigan researchers found that a sense of fitting in was more important to good health than the number of friends and acquaintances one maintains.

Making It Real

It's not so easy to get connected in our culture—it takes a conscious effort to attain it. "Our whole society is set up for the most part to keep us separate and alone, so we're not dependent on anyone else," says Carolyn Shaffer, the author of *Creating Community Anywhere: Finding Support and Connection in a Fragmented World.*

In pondering ways to expand your personal connections, look at the ones you already have, suggests Shaffer. "You might be more connected than you think."

Recall the people you really enjoy being with. Then to end a sense of fragmentation in your own social life, bring those friends and family together. She suggests that, rather than having people mill about at a party, give the group a focus, at least at some stage during the event. For example, at a birthday party, gather the group as the cake is served and focus all the attention on the person being celebrated, perhaps sharing stories about the person.

Small things, like regular emails or brief phone calls with friends or family, can also create satisfying connections. Shaffer and a friend leave a voice mail for each other every evening, describing one thing they were grateful for that day. "It's the tiniest thing," she says. "But you make it regular, and it can then go deeper."

Join what she calls "affinity groups," like walking, gardening or book clubs. Strong bonds and even friendships often spring from those. "If you can't find one that works for you, start one," she adds. Churches often provide this sense of community and support as well.

There's also a powerful and practical group gathering called a "brain exchange," Shaffer says. Participants usually meet monthly, and those attending can present a question, ranging from business concerns like a hiring decision, a potential job move or how to ask for a raise, to personal questions like planning a vacation, buying a new computer, or handling a difficult relationship.

"Brainstorming rules" are followed, and each question-and-answer session is kept to about 10 minutes. Shaffer has attended one for years, and says the exchanges "have turned people's lives around." In addition, you get a chance to be a resource to others. "The giving is as important as receiving," she notes.

To Learn More

Visit the WebMD site at www.webmd.com. In the Search box, type in "social connections," "friendship" or "marriage" for studies on these topics.

CHAPTER 10

Lend a Hand

Nature guide, mentor, museum docent, and inner-city tutor.

What do all of these people have in common? They're volunteers, and studies show they're living longer and more satisfying lives as a result. In fact, regularly volunteering one's services to others is among the most powerful means of warding off premature death, according to numerous studies.

But before you dial up your local volunteer center, know that some volunteer activities are better than others. And you don't want to push yourself too hard; that undoes all the health benefits and may just burn you out.

What Scientists Know

It's the act of giving, not simply the sociability of volunteer activities, that imparts life-enhancing benefits, says Stephanie Brown, PhD, a psychologist with the Institute for Social Research at the University of Michigan. In a 2003 study, Brown reported that the risk of premature death among study participants during a five-year period declined by more than half, compared with "non-givers." The "givers" in the study were people 65 years and older who regularly volunteered to help others with errands, housekeeping, transportation, babysitting and other tasks.

Scientists strongly suspect that the act of giving triggers the release of pleasure-inducing brain chemicals called endorphins, creating a "helper's high." Providing valuable assistance to others also gives rise to feelings of pride, satisfaction and enjoyment, which counteract the stress- and depression-inducing effects of negative emotions.

"People feeling positive emotions recover more quickly from stress," Brown says. "You can imagine where helping over your lifetime is beneficial by helping to buffer the effects of stress." Other researchers point out that volunteering also improves one's sense of self worth, and gives a sense of "being somebody."

What's intriguing about Brown's research is that it shows that in the usual give-and-take of relationships, those on the giving end get the most health benefits. Brown found that people who receive much more support than they give actually had a slightly higher risk of early death, even after factoring in the effect of the physical health of both parties.

Making It Real

Since you can choose from a host of activities, think carefully before signing on for a volunteer project. It should, of course, be a job you'll enjoy. Ideally, it will even be slightly exhilarating.

In addition, volunteer for activities that put you in direct contact with people. It's those close, personal activities that really provide the emotional rewards.

Consistency also matters. You'll get the most benefits by volunteering regularly, at least one hour a week. But be careful about burning out. Some organizations may have such demands for volunteers that their needs begin to tax you. If you begin to feel resentful, guilty for saying no to volunteering, or stressed about your obligations, it's time to step back. You should only be getting pleasure from volunteering. "Give to the point that it feels good and stop after that," says Brown.

Another key point to keep in mind: If you're in a one-on-one relationship in a volunteer activity—like visiting an elderly person or tutoring a child—work to foster independence and self-respect in the person you're assisting. If the relationship becomes one of excessive dependence on you, it's not good for either party.

To Learn More

Point your browser to www.volunteermatch.org to learn about volunteer activities in your region. Type in your zip code for a list of nearby opportunities.

You can also look in the Yellow Pages. Check out the "Volunteering" heading in the index, or flip to the "Social and Human Services" section.

CHAPTER 11

Take Time for Tea

When patriots at the Boston Tea Party in 1773 dumped shipments of green and black tea into Boston Harbor's cold waters, they might have held onto some of the chests had they understood tea's potent health benefits.

At the time, tea was the most popular beverage in the world, next to water. More green tea than black was actually consumed then in Europe—with black tea rising to its current popularity in Western culture only in the late 19th century.

Europeans loved tea for its flavor and for the elegant ritual of tea service. But for thousands of years, the Chinese had revered tea for a different reason: its health benefits. Over the past few decades, scientists have been taking a closer look at the brew, and have come to similar conclusions. Study after study in both animals and humans demonstrate an ever-growing list of the disease-preventing properties of the polyphenols found in tea. These plant compounds are nature's way to protect plants from external and internal assaults, and appear to do the same for humans. As one doctor put it, maybe a bottle of this brew belongs in the medicine chest.

What Scientists Know

A leading authority on tea and health, John H. Weisburger, MD, PhD, drinks about eight cups of tea a day, most of it black tea, for its myriad of health benefits. He recommends drinking between five and ten cups a day. "One or two cups a day doesn't do a thing," Weisburger says.

All varieties of tea (not to be confused with herbal infusions, which are often incorrectly called teas) come from the leaves of the same plant—Camellia sinensis. The essential differences between types of tea, whether green, oolong, or black, arise from the level of processing the leaves undergo after picking. Green, which is dried and then steamed, receives the least processing. Black tea receives the most, and oolong gets an intermediate amount. Because of its minimal processing, green tea retains the polyphenol called EGCG, the powerful antioxidant that gives green tea its superstar status.

Green tea currently gets most of the acclaim, as black tea hasn't been studied as extensively, Weisburger says. In conducting side-by-side comparisons of both teas, he found they provide similar health benefits. Weisburger points out that in the processing of black tea, EGCG is just converted to a different, but still powerful, antioxidant.

The ability to tame free radicals gives tea its powerful health punch. These unstable molecules, normal by-products of metabolism, do their damage by grabbing electrons from DNA and other cellular material. Most, but not all, of the harm done by free radicals is repaired by the body. The damage accumulates in the body, potentially triggering cancer, heart disease, immune system decline, brain dysfunction, and cataracts.

The polyphenols in tea are rich in antioxidants, the "free radical scavengers" that help protect the body. Regular tea consumption keeps these antioxidants circulating, where they block free radical formation and activity.

Recent studies show that tea plays a role in the prevention of heart attacks and strokes. Tea's antioxidants inhibit blood platelets from sticking together to form deadly clots, and the antioxidants also prevent the oxidation of LDL cholesterol, a critical step in plaque formation.

Regularly drinking tea may be among the best cancer-fighting strategies you can adopt. The lowest prostate cancer rates in the world are in China and Japan, where green tea is widely consumed. The rate of esophageal cancer, which is often triggered by smoking, is 60 percent lower in smokers who also drink green tea.

Women with early-stage breast cancer had lower rates of remission when they drank at least eight cups of tea a day. High levels of tea consumption were also correlated with lower levels of breast cancer in a study of almost 9,000 Japanese women. Recent research with tea also shows encouraging results against stomach, pancreas, colon and lung cancers. Topical treatments with green tea showed impressive protection against skin cancer with lab animals. Mayo Clinic researchers recently found that green tea kills off leukemia cells in adults, with no toxic side effects.

Tea also appears to boost the immune system by prompting immune cells to more aggressively attack microbial invaders. A recent study found that EGCG in green tea disrupts the binding of HIV to human T cells, the initial step in HIV infection. Studies also report that tea significantly ameliorates inflammatory conditions like arthritis and gout, and even lowers rates of gum disease.

Making It Real

Tea contains about 50 mg of caffeine per cup, compared with the 130 mg found in coffee. Decaf tea is widely available, but studies indicate it loses some of its cancer-protection properties. And if you're a coffee lover, you don't need to kick the habit, just switch to tea at some point during the day.

If you want to really get a dose of the beneficial tea compounds, look for the rare and somewhat expensive white tea, which contains even greater concentrations of the principal polyphenol ECGC.

Tea should be brewed four to five minutes to ensure maximum infusion of the beneficial compounds. For maximum benefit, you should also drink tea throughout the day. Jeffrey Blumberg, PhD, a professor of nutrition and chief of the Antioxidants Research Lab at the Jean Mayer USDA Human Nutrition Research Center on Aging in Boston, explains that the bloodstream can only absorb the beneficial compounds in about one cup of tea, which circulates for about an hour before passing from the body. So to maintain adequate circulating levels of tea's healthful compounds, you'll need to sip it throughout the day.

Finally, forget about bottled teas, as their levels of polyphenols are essentially nil, due to processing and the fact that tea polyphenols degrade within a few hours of brewing.

To Learn More

Visit the Tea Association of the United States of America's website at www.teausa.com.

CHAPTER 12

Shed Your Stress

Your boss, an overbearing man who frequently berates workers, approaches your desk. Your body tenses and your breathing turns shallow as you brace to explain why your report isn't finished.

You're on the freeway, dialing your cell phone to let your wife know you'll be late to dinner and you catch part of the radio report that says there's a crash in the tech stocks. Then your pager sounds.

At home, a stack of unpaid bills lies on your desk. Just looking at them ties your stomach in a knot as you ponder your depleted bank account.

Millions of scenarios like these play out daily, making stress an almost constant companion for legions of people while sapping their health and enjoyment of life.

But lest stress earn a uniformly bad reputation, keep in mind that humanity couldn't have survived without it. How else could our ancient ancestors, when suddenly confronted with a saber-toothed tiger or an enemy warrior, have instantly marshaled the mental acuity and physical strength to fight or flee for their lives? And stress is still valuable in modern times, like giving you sharpness and focus during a job interview, while taking an exam, or when running to catch an airplane.

"We have a term for stressors that are mild to moderate and that don't last for too long," says Robert Sapolsky, PhD, a renowned stress expert from Stanford University. "We call them stimulation. We don't aim for a life without stress; we aim for a life with just the right amount."

What Scientists Know

Think of stress as your body's response to something that challenges your sense of well being. There are two kinds of stress: physical stress, for example, from a bodily injury, and psychological stress, the kind that causes most of our health problems and is our focus.

Stress starts in the brain with a thought or perception. When you perceive something as a threat to your well being, your mind directs the release of adrenaline and cortisol. These hormones then trigger a cascade of additional hormones. It's stress response that heightens mental alertness, increases the heart rate to speed more oxygen and glucose to muscles, and shortens breath. This process also temporarily boosts the immune system to fight infections from a potential injury while slowing long-term growth activities like bone formation in order to divert resources to address the immediate crisis.

"It's very useful for moderate, transient stressors where you actually have to be thinking clearly at the time," says Sapolsky. But after a few hours, "it's just sheer bad news, because you can't always be on an emergency economy."

While the first surge of the stress hormone cortisol sharpens thinking, it does the opposite when chronically circulating. Cortisol in the brain interferes with concentration, impairs memory and, if levels are high enough, even kills brain cells. Some researchers now suspect that this explains the dementia-like symptoms experienced by a growing number of people in their thirties and forties, whose multitasking lives keep them in constant overdrive.

Chronic stress can also elevate blood pressure and damage the cardiovascular system, giving rise to heart disease and stroke. A 2004 study from University of California, San Francisco grabbed headlines with its findings that chronic stress can speed the death of cells, causing premature aging.

Muscles initially energized by stress eventually become fatigued. The stress-induced demand for glucose can trigger diabetes. Stress-stalled bone formation can cause osteoporosis. Stress even dampens libido.

Numerous other serious health conditions are linked to stress: insomnia, arthritis, and some cancers, among other diseases. Stress triggers or worsens anxiety, depression, and panic disorders. Chronic stress depresses the immune system, leaving people more vulnerable to autoimmune disorders, incipient cancers, and contagious illnesses such as colds and influenza.

Making It Real

Before you despair at this daunting litany of stress-induced ailments, keep in mind that the level of stress you endure often lies largely in your hands.

The attitude you adopt toward an unwelcome outcome or event is pivotal to eliminating stress from your life. Putting a disappointment or perceived threat in context can help you see it's not worth getting upset over, in the grand scheme.

People who live to age 100 and older are a living testimony to that philosophy. They're what researchers term "stress shedders." These calm elders seem to shrug off setbacks that can annoy or even devastate others.

Cultivating a strong group of friends is a bulwark against chronic stress. "In terms of stress-reducing interventions, probably the one which overall is most impressive is the effect of social connections, social support," Sapolsky says.

You can exercise stress away as well. Stress experts like Sapolsky regularly work out to reduce tension. Simply walking for 30 minutes a day can make a dramatic difference in lowering stress levels.

Try meditating. Studies show it's a very effective way to control stress. When confronted with a stressful situation, use deep breathing to relax. In addition, give up multi-tasking. Studies show it creates unnecessary stress and the "efficiency gains" are illusory.

Psychotherapy is also a proven stress reliever. Consider visiting a mental health professional if you're enduring high stress levels. Many insurers also pay for stress management seminars.

Other tips on living a low-stress life: practice better planning and organization; learn to say no to demanding people; simplify your life, and be judicious in the use of electronic communication tools, which often just keep you working at all hours rather than improving productivity; and count to 10 before responding to people when you're angry.

To Learn More

Visit the U.S. Centers for Disease Control and Prevention's stress-related website at www.cdc.gov/niosh/topics/stress. The site includes an online booklet called "Stress, At Work," which you can print. The booklet can also be ordered, at no charge, by calling (800) 356-4674.

The American Psychological Association offers a free brochure called "The Road to Resilience." Order it by calling (800) 964-2000, or downloading an online version on the Association's "Help Center" at http://helping.apa.org. The site also offers advice on meeting life's challenges.

CHAPTER 13

Get Physical

Ever since Jack La Lanne hit the airwaves in 1951, the "Godfather of Fitness" has been exhorting Americans to get off their couches and enjoy the active life.

His plain and direct advice has remained unchanged through the decades: There are no quick fixes to fitness. It takes dedication, but the payoffs are tremendous.

"Your health account is like your bank account. The more you put in, the more you can take out," La Lanne states emphatically in a video clip on his website. "The only way you can hurt the body is don't use it."

La Lanne has become a living testament to his philosophy. At age 90, he still works out two hours a day—one hour swimming and one hour with weights—and exudes the vitality of a man decades younger.

But he wasn't always a paragon of fitness. As a youth, he routinely gorged in sugary foods, and became moody, hostile, and at one point suicidal. Then his life changed after he went to a talk on healthful living. "I just changed a few bad habits, replaced them with good habits, and the whole life changed," he says. "That's when it started, then I was so caught up with physical fitness." That good habit of exercise that he so enthusiastically adopted decades ago turns out to help prevent just about every age-related chronic condition.

What Scientists Know

If a pill could deliver all the benefits of exercise, people would pay dearly to get it. Exercise strengthens the heart muscle and reduces the risk of heart attacks and strokes. By dilating blood vessels, it helps lower blood pressure. Physical activity improves blood cholesterol profiles, and helps prevents arterial plaque buildup and the aggregation of blood platelets, both of which can form dangerous blood clots. One study of 73,000 women found those briskly walking for 30 minutes a day cut their risk of a heart attack by up to 40 percent. In another study of 11,000 men, those who walked briskly for 30 minutes, 5 days a week, cut their stroke risk by a quarter. Those walking double that amount halved their stroke risk.

Regular exercise strengthens bones by mildly stressing them. Research shows both men and women who exercise have denser bones and are less likely to develop osteoporosis.

Moderate to vigorous exercise improves insulin's ability to deliver sugar to the cells, and can cut the risk of Type 1 diabetes by almost half. It can even reduce diabetics' need for medication, according to other research.

By working out, you markedly reduce your chances of getting cancers of the breast and prostate by modulating the effects of hormones that promote tumor development. Exercise also protects against colon cancer, possibly by decreasing gastrointestinal transit time. And if this isn't convincing enough, physical activity lifts you emotionally and mentally. Exercise fights stress and anxiety, and in some cases works as well as medication and psychotherapy for depression. Exercisers even appear to retain more gray matter as they age, according to recent research. This may explain why studies have found that exercisers have superior memory and thinking skills, compared to the sedentary. There's even evidence that physically active people have a lower risk for Alzheimer's disease. Regular exercise also improves self-esteem and helps you get a good night's sleep.

It's easier to maintain an ideal body weight with exercise. Regular physical exertion increases your resting metabolic rate, which causes you to burn more calories even at rest.

Making It Real

It's not easy to develop a regular exercise program, nor is it always fun. Even La Lanne says he really doesn't enjoy exercising, but hasn't missed a daily workout in 75 years.

He likes the results, he says, such as his 31" waist. It all boils down to willpower, La Lanne stresses.

Fortunately, you don't necessarily need a La Lanne routine. The American College of Sports Medicine reports that 3 to 5 workouts weekly, of 30 to 60 minutes each, deliver the vast majority of the health benefits.

However, Jeffrey Potteiger, PhD, chair of the Department of Physical Education at Miami University in Ohio, doesn't want to scare people off from regular exercise even with those figures. "We now know that if you become a little bit active you're going to get some sort of benefit," Potteiger says. "What you want to do is get people started and get them hooked."

Potteiger counsels those short on time to fit shorter bouts of physical activity into their schedule, such as a 10-minute walk in the morning, a short walk at lunch, and another in the evening. "All of a sudden you've got 30 to 40 minutes of exercise, and that's a lot better than doing nothing."

However, if possible, it's best to get a continuous workout for at least 30 minutes. In general, the higher the level of intensity you achieve, and the longer the duration, the more fitness benefits you accrue, Potteiger says. And discard the tired and dangerous adage: "No pain, no gain." If you feel pain, you're injuring yourself.

You're also never too old to start a fitness program, although you have to be more cautious the older you get, Potteiger says. Anyone older than 65 years, or with a risk factor for heart disease, should get a physical checkup before starting.

You do need some degree of exertion, like briskly walking, running, swimming, or bike riding, to maximize the health benefits. Activities like dancing, gardening, or housecleaning are also valuable, Potteiger notes, because they burn calories and maintain some level of fitness. However, they generally don't provide the same level of fitness benefit as sustained aerobic or strength training exercise.

To Learn More

Visit the National Institutes of Health's website on exercise and physical fitness at www.nlm.nih.gov/medlineplus/exerciseandphysicalfitness.html. The site provides information, studies and links to other websites related to physical fitness. Also visit the website for the President's Council on Physical Fitness and Sport at www.fitness.gov.

CHAPTER **14**

Join the Resistance

For decades, weight training was the stepchild in the family of exercise. The health benefits were rarely investigated by mainstream medicine or covered by the popular press. The value seemed only recognized by devotees pumping iron in health clubs or by the hunks at places like Venice Beach.

"It was only thought if you were an athlete that you need to do strength training," says Jeffrey Potteiger, PhD, chair of the Department of Physical Education at Miami University in Ohio. "We've come to realize that people need cardiovascular fitness *and* strength."

And truly turning old thinking on its head, researchers now realize that strength training actually becomes more crucial with age. "You could make the argument that it's more important for an older adult to maintain strength than cardiovascular fitness," Potteiger says. "At the very least, it's just as important."

The reason? Besides conferring virtually all the benefits we associate with exercise, there's no activity that so effectively slows the body's dismaying shift from muscle to flab. In the absence of resistance training, research shows that after age 40, we lose up to a third of a pound of muscle a year. By age 70, you may have lost 25 percent or more of your muscle mass if you haven't exercised. The mobility and strength taken for granted as a youth can become just a memory.

What Scientists Know

Irwin Rosenberg, MD, a senior scientist with the Human Nutrition Research Center on Aging at Tufts University, gave a name to the gradual muscle wasting so closely linked to old age. He called it "sarcopenia," which means "vanishing flesh" in Greek.

Rosenberg says loss of muscle strength is a key factor—in addition to bone loss—behind crippling hip fractures in older people. He also believes that many of the people now reliant on walkers and wheelchairs could have avoided that fate had they known to strength train earlier in their lives.

Resistance training increases concentrations of growth-promoting agents, particularly human growth hormone, testosterone, and insulin. Together they increase uptake of glucose, carbohydrates, and amino acids from blood into the muscle, increasing muscle mass. They also stimulate protein synthesis in bone and cartilage.

With weight training, a group of seniors on average gained three pounds of muscle and lost four pounds of fat after only three months. Their resting metabolism also increased by seven percent, boosting their daily caloric burn by 15 percent.

A Harvard University study of more than 44,000 men linked regular weight training with a one-third reduction in their risk of developing cardiovascular disease. It can also help control diabetes, ease the pain of arthritis, and improve balance. The role of weight training in strengthening bones is well documented, and, when done correctly, it can even relieve lower back pain.

In a landmark study at Tufts University, nine frail nursing home residents—with the youngest aged 86—found their muscle strength increased an average of 175 percent with two months of weight training. A 2004 study revealed that not only can the very elderly work out with light weights, but they can safely get better results with a more challenging weight routine.

Strength training can also rev up your outlook. Studies show it can ameliorate depression as effectively as medication. And the mental lift and increased physical strength it provides energizes people to become more confident and active in all aspects of life. It can also help you sleep better.

Making It Real

The best advice before embarking on a weight-training program is to take it easy. And always check with your doctor prior to starting any exercise program if you're over age 65 or have a chronic health condition or a risk factor for heart disease, like excess weight.

Advice varies on how many repetitions of each type of weight-bearing exercise, called a set, that you should complete. The President's Council on Physical Fitness and Sports states that for older adults, a single set of 10 to 15 repetitions of 8 to 10 different types of exercise provides an adequate amount of training for both muscular strength and endurance when performed 2 to 3 times a week.

"It's better than doing nothing and probably appropriate," says Potteiger of the one-set recommendation, particularly for older people. "But if you do a little more, you'll then get stronger, faster."

Because proper technique is important to maximize gains and avoid strains, the American College of Sports Medicine advises beginners to work on weight machines, since machines control the range of movement and help prevent incorrect postures.

It's important to vary your routine, adds Potteiger. "You want to give the tissues of the body different kinds of stimulus. If all you're doing is the same repetitions, that stimulus will no longer give results." So change intensity, or periodically alternate between machines and free weights. But be careful of overexertion. If you feel pain, stop, because you're injuring yourself.

A word of advice to running, biking, or walking aficionados: as valuable as they are for maintaining robust health, they're unfortunately not enough to prevent the steady loss of muscle with age, particularly in the upper body. To do that, you also need to pump some iron.

And women need have no fear about bulking up from strength training. It requires lots of testosterone to make that happen, and women just don't have enough. Strength training instead makes women's bodies firmer and better defined.

Be sure to stretch when your workout is finished. Moving your body through a full range of motion ensures flexibility and ameliorates muscular discomfort.

To Learn More

Visit the American College of Sports Medicine's website at www.acsm.org. Click on the "Health & Fitness Information" icon on the home page.

Visit the CDC's Nutrition and Physical Activity Program website at www.cdc.gov/nccdphp/dnpa/index.htm. Scroll down to the heading "Growing Stronger: Strength Training for Older Adults" for detailed information on strength training.

CHAPTER 15

Keep Your Arteries Clean

Heart disease and stroke—the first and third causes of death in the United States—share a common origin. They both arise from unhealthy arteries, with walls clogged by hard deposits called plaque. As plaque accumulates, it constricts blood flow to the heart or brain. Plaque can then break off, blocking arteries and triggering a sudden heart attack or stroke.

Roughly one million Americans die of cardiovascular disease each year. More than 60 million Americans have some form of cardiovascular disease, according to the Centers for Disease Control and Prevention.

But this isn't part of nature's plan. Heart disease and strokes aren't inevitable consequences of aging. In Japan, for example, where people eat less red meat and get more exercise, cardiovascular disease isn't nearly as common.

Staying free of heart disease and stroke requires keeping your arteries—part of your body's plumbing system—healthy, elastic and free of plaque. The choices you make in what you eat, your level of physical activity and the weight you maintain largely determines how well you achieve this crucial health goal.

What Scientists Know

The human heart, a muscle the size of a large fist, pumps oxygenated blood into arteries that extend throughout the body. The heart, like all muscles, needs a blood supply to fuel itself. That's supplied by the coronary artery. The carotid artery sends blood to the brain. When plaque begins to accumulate in arteries, a condition called atherosclerosis, there's trouble. When the coronary artery becomes blocked, a heart attack occurs. When the carotid artery is blocked, a stroke results.

So what causes plaque accumulation on arterial walls? In short, it's the nature of your blood chemistry and the level of your blood pressure. In simplest terms, blood chemistry refers to the myriad of compounds circulating in blood, including cholesterol, triglycerides, homocysteine, cortisol, and C-reactive protein. Blood pressure, the force blood exerts against arterial walls, profoundly influences cardiovascular health, since excess pressure irritates the walls, triggering plaque buildup.

Cholesterol, despite its bad reputation, is essential in building cell membranes and manufacturing hormones. Nature has devised a two-part transport system cholesterol: via LDLs and HDLs. Low-density lipoproteins

(LDLs) act as vehicles, carrying cholesterol from the liver to "job sites" in the body where it's needed. High-density lipoproteins (HDLs) on the other hand, shuttle excess cholesterol—including that accumulated in plaque—back to the liver for reprocessing. Despite its good works, LDL cholesterol is also the potential troublemaker. At high concentrations, or when they become oxidized, LDLs can damage arterial walls. This damage can cause plaque accumulation.

But cholesterol is far from the sole villain behind cardiovascular disease, since about half of people dying from plugged-up arteries have normal levels. Other blood factors play key roles. Triglycerides, which mainly come from animal products and saturated fats, are fat molecules circulating in blood. High levels can interfere with normal functioning of arteries and encourage plaque buildup. Homocysteine is emerging as another key player in heart health. The amino acid, which comes from animal protein, can irritate artery walls at elevated levels, according to studies. Excess weight seriously compromises heart health, as it raises levels of tryglycerides and LDL. It also strains the heart and can elevate blood pressure. Cortisol, the hormone released in response to stress, also triggers heart damage, mainly by elevating blood pressure.

The American Heart Association has also recently identified elevated levels of C-reactive protein—a sign of inflammation—as a risk factor for cardiovascular disease. And combined with high blood pressure, elevated CRP levels increase stroke and heart attack risk up to eightfold, according to a 2003 study.

That's the grim news. But you've got much control over how healthy your pipes—and hence your cardiovascular system—remain throughout your life. What's the top priority? That's simple: Exercise. Research shows physical activity reduces blood pressure, maintains crucial arterial elasticity, lowers stress hormones, and improves the ratio of HDL to LDL cholesterols while lowering overall levels. Exercise, of course, also keeps weight in check.

A diet high in fruits, vegetables, whole grains, and nuts runs a close second. They provide antioxidants that help prevent LDL oxidation. They contain fiber, which aids in clearing fats and cholesterol from the body. They deliver minerals essential to heart health, like magnesium and potassium. These foods are also rich in B-vitamins and folic acid, which help to break down homocysteine.

Aspirin improves blood chemistry. Small, regular doses can prevent blood platelet aggregation and reduce arterial wall inflammation, which can rupture plaque, sending it into the bloodstream and potentially blocking an artery.

Omega-3 fatty acids found in fish like salmon, sardines and trout also appear to moderate platelet clumping and tame arterial inflammation. Wine consumed in moderation (one drink a day for women, and one to two for men) also provides significant heart health benefits. Studies show that wine and other spirits can help prevent blood clot development and increase HDL levels.

Making It Real

The best advice for preventing heart disease follows a familiar refrain: Stay physically active and nourish your body with foods that promote good blood chemistry, and, consequently, good heart health.

It's difficult, if not impossible, to keep your cardiovascular system healthy if you're carrying excess weight. Everyone knows that by now. The challenge is getting weight off, and keeping it off. You simply must exercise to have any hope of achieving heart health and an optimal weight. Take a clue from cardiologists, who as a rule regularly work out. It needn't be difficult. Walking is an excellent exercise, and it's convenient, pleasant, and conducive to creative thinking.

Go easy with animal-based foods, like meat, eggs, and dairy products, in your diet. Americans eat way too much, and it's the chief source of excess cholesterol, homocysteine and triglycerides. It's easier to do than you think.

If you're in a high risk category for heart disease, you should talk with your doctor about using aspirin to prevent a heart attack.

To Learn More

Become familiar with the American Heart Association's website, at www.heart.org. Also, visit the Centers for Disease Control and Prevention's site on heart disease prevention at www.cdc.gov/nccdphp/bb_heartdisease.htm.

CHAPTER 16

Halt Hypertension

One of the most chilling aspects of hypertension is how quietly it does its damage. There are usually no outward signs of trouble, but it can make itself known in devastating ways. Heart attacks, strokes, blindness, kidney failure, aneurysms, and even dementia can be caused by tissues slowly damaged by chronically high blood pressure.

Hypertension, or high blood pressure, is the most prevalent cardiovascular disease in America. A staggering 65 million Americans have hypertension, and yet less than one-third realize it. Another 45 million have a recently identified condition called "pre-hypertension."

Because of its prevalence, hypertension is often viewed as an inevitable part of aging, much like gray hair. "That's definitely a myth," states Paul K. Whelton, MD, MSc, an authority on hypertension and a professor at Tulane University in New Orleans. The vast majority of cases are "completely preventable" with proper diet and lifestyle. People in Eastern cultures, like India and China, largely remain hypertension-free their entire lives, he says, until "they become Westernized."

What Scientists Know

When the powerful heart muscle contracts, it pumps a surge of blood into the arteries, momentarily raising pressure inside the vascular system. In the pause between contractions, the pressure drops. A normal reading is less than 120 mm Hg as the heart contracts (systolic pressure) and less than 80 mm Hg at rest (diastolic pressure). Levels between 120 and 139 mm Hg systolic and 80 and 89 mm Hg diastolic are now called pre-hypertension. Those with pre-hypertension are at significant risk of developing hypertension and its complications. Levels of 140/90 and above are designated hypertension.

A blood pressure reading tells a story about the state of your cardiovascular system. Normal arteries expand and contract, like flexible hoses, to accommodate increases and decreases in blood flow. But when arteries become "hardened" by plaque accumulation, the pressure rises within them as the heart struggles to deliver the same amount of blood through the constricted tubes. In addition, hypertension also arises when the thin muscle layers, which line arteries and control their contraction and expansion, thicken or malfunction.

Hypertension strains the heart, which can cause it to enlarge and increase the risk of heart failure.

Hypertension also triples heart attack risk, Whelton says. Stroke risk multiplies with increasing blood pressure, up to tenfold in those with severe cases. Pressure damage to blood vessels in the kidneys, eyes and brain can lead to kidney failure, damaged eyesight, and cognitive impairment.

Fortunately, hypertension responds to healthful lifestyle changes. Experts agree that losing excess weight is the single most important measure for lowering blood pressure rates. A three-year study found that just a 10-pound loss significantly lowered blood pressure. Exercise also has a strong influence. A 2004 study of adults with hypertension linked 10 weeks of moderate aerobic workouts with a blood pressure drop of 13 mm Hg. Chronic stress is another hypertension trigger. Stress reduction measures, like meditation and stress management training, can lower blood pressure; in one recent study by 6 mm Hg.

Diet profoundly affects blood pressure. Salt is a leading culprit behind high blood pressure, a result of the body's effort to eliminate excess sodium. The average American consumes at least 10,000 milligrams a day of salt, and one study found that reducing that daily intake by 3,000 milligrams lowered blood pressure on average 10 mm Hg. This decline cuts risk of stroke death by one-fifth and heart disease mortality by one-sixth.

A low-sodium diet that's high in fruits, vegetables, low-fat dairy products, and omega-3 fatty acids, while low on saturated fats, makes a dramatic difference in blood pressure levels. A recent study of people with hypertension who followed this diet for a month reported that participants' pressure dropped on average 11.5 mm Hg, compared with those following a typical American diet. Minerals like calcium, magnesium and especially potassium also play crucial functions in maintaining normal blood pressure. An analysis of 33 studies found increased potassium intake linked with an average 4.4 mm Hg drop in blood pressure in those with hypertension. And vitamin D deficiencies are also linked to hypertension, perhaps due to the vitamin's role in controlling renin, a hormone that regulates blood pressure.

Making It Real

Where do you begin in preventing high blood pressure, or lowering it? Lose excess weight. "Absolutely that should be the first step," says Whelton. Also, lose weight slowly, around two to four pounds per month, as sudden drops can exacerbate hypertension.

Get moving to keep blood pressure under control. Exercise will not only help you lose weight, but will improve the health of your heart and vascular system. Whelton's research shows that regularity is more important than intensity with exercise. Just walking several times a week can significantly lower blood pressure, he says.

Add salt sparingly to your food, if at all, and cultivate a taste for doing without it. While health officials suggest consuming no more than 6,000 mg a day of salt, people can safely function with far less, down to about 1,200 mg a day. Unprocessed fruits, vegetables, meat, and fish actually provide all the sodium you need.

If only to lower blood pressure, it's crucial to fit more fruits and vegetables into your diet. And limit consumption of red meat while enjoying fish at least two to three times a week. Be certain you're getting at least recommended daily intakes of essential minerals and vitamins.

Throw out your cigarettes. Just one can temporarily raise blood pressure by as much as 10 points. If you drink, keep it to no more than two a day, as any amount beyond that can elevate blood pressure.

Medications can also effectively control hypertension. However, they have sometimes serious side effects. When hypertension isn't acute, Whelton suggests giving diet and lifestyle changes a few months before taking medication. But in the end, do whatever is necessary to keep blood pressure under control.

To Learn More

Visit the National Heart, Lung, and Blood Institute's website, "Your Guide to Lowering High Blood Pressure" at www.nhlbi.nih.gov/hbp. You can also call the NHLBI's Health Information Center at (301) 592-8573 to request information about hypertension.

CHAPTER 17

Dodge Diabetes

These days, insulin has a tough time doing its job. This hormone plays the essential role of escorting blood sugar molecules to cells and then ushering them inside, where they're converted into energy. But due to an insidious complex of reactions—most tied to excess weight, poor diets, and a lack of physical activity—cells begin to close their doors to insulin and thus blood sugar. Then the pancreas, which produces insulin, works overtime to make more, in a largely vain attempt to knock harder at the cell doors. Eventually, the pancreas wears down from this extra effort, and insulin production lags. Meanwhile, sugar, or glucose, accumulates in the blood like a poison, damaging nerves and blood vessels throughout the body and causing complications ranging from heart disease, stroke, blindness, and kidney disease to nerve degeneration that can require amputation of limbs. Those enduring this disorder also often cope with bouts of fatigue and depression.

This is Type 2 diabetes, which accounts for at least 90 percent of all diabetes cases and is predominantly linked to lifestyle choices. About 18 million Americans have it. Another 40 million are estimated to have "pre-diabetes," or impaired glucose tolerance, in which insulin resistance is building in cells and baseline blood sugar levels are rising. (About 10 percent of Americans have Type 1 diabetes, either a genetic or infectious disorder caused by an autoimmune reaction or a viral infection, and which destroys the pancreas' ability to produce insulin.)

Type 2 diabetes rates are rising. The Centers for Disease Control and Prevention states that children born today now have at least a one in three chance of developing this debilitating disease in their lifetime. Adults diagnosed at age 40 carve off at least 12 years of life expectancy due to the disease, according to the CDC.

What Scientists Know

Years of research shows that diabetes is one of the most preventable of the chronic diseases plaguing Americans. By far the most important step is losing excess weight, which has a strong effect in reducing blood sugar levels while maintaining or improving the insulin sensitivity of cells.

Even modest weight loss, combined with regular exercise, makes a dramatic difference, according to a federally sponsored 2002 study. Researchers running that study, called the Diabetes Prevention Program, recruited 3,234 adults with pre-diabetes. During a three-year period, participants who exercised 30 minutes a day, five days a week, and ate a low-calorie, low-fat diet, lost an average of 15 pounds. That dropped their odds of progressing to full diabetes by a stunning 58 percent.

What surprised health experts was the degree of protection provided by such modest weight loss, which was on average 5 to 7 percent of body weight. A 160-pound woman only needs to lose about 10 pounds and engage in regular physical activity like walking to achieve the sharp risk reduction, the study reported.

Moderate weight training can also help to prevent or control diabetes, studies show. Building skeletal muscle improves insulin sensitivity and increases the uptake of blood glucose. Sleep deprivation is also linked to insulin resistance and diabetes onset. In one study, healthy young adults getting 4 hours of sleep per night for six nights temporarily entered a pre-diabetic state, recovering when their sleep deficit was restored. Chronic stress is also associated with diabetes, both because people under stress may indulge in unhealthful eating patterns and because stress hormones have a direct effect on blood glucose levels, according to the American Diabetes Association.

The types of food you eat also influence your risk of developing diabetes. High fiber foods, like whole grains, vegetables, and fruits, slow down the uptake of glucose, easing the workload on cellular energy factories. In contrast, foods like white bread, white rice, soft drinks, and french fries were associated with increases in the rates of diabetes. Foods containing "good fats," like omega-3 fatty acids, improve the health of cell membranes—which are largely composed of fats—by increasing their receptivity to insulin. In addition, replacing trans-fatty acids with polyunsaturated fats reduced the risk of developing diabetes by 40 percent in one study. Light drinking is also associated with a lowered incidence of diabetes, as it improves cells' sensitivity to insulin (although heavy drinking appears to do the opposite). The authors of a 2004 study on lifestyle and diabetes concluded that "a healthy diet, together with regular physical activity, maintenance of a healthy weight, moderate alcohol consumption, and avoidance of sedentary behaviors and smoking could nearly eliminate Type 2 diabetes." However, they add, "there is a still a wide gap between what we know and what we practice."

Making It Real

In addition to adopting the lifestyle described above, people should monitor their blood glucose levels, as diabetes shows few outward symptoms until permanent damage is underway. Cathy Tibbetts, a certified diabetes educator with American Diabetes Association, says those with risk factors for diabetes, like a family history or anyone over age 45 with body mass index over 25, should have their blood glucose tested. While most doctors automatically request a glucose test when ordering a routine blood test, Tibbetts advises people to verify that one was ordered. She also says that the American Diabetes Association encourages people to become active consumers and ask for the results of their blood tests.

If it tests normal for glucose, then continue to monitor your blood sugar levels every three years, Tibbetts says. However, if the test shows you have pre-diabetes, you should get a yearly glucose test, she says, while immediately launching lifestyle changes to prevent it from advancing to diabetes.

To Learn More

Visit the Center's for Disease Control and Prevention's Diabetes Prevention website at www.ndep.nih.gov/diabetes/prev/prevention.htm. You can order the CDC's free publication, "Am I at Risk for Type 2 Diabetes?" by calling (800) 860-8747. Also, visit the American Diabetes Association's website at www.diabetes.org. Look for its "Diabetes Risk Test" to assess your odds of developing diabetes.

CHAPTER 18

Prevent Colon Cancer

Colon cancer doesn't quite garner the attention as other types of cancer, although it should. It's the second leading cause of cancer deaths in men and women combined in the United States, behind lung cancer. About 150,000 people are diagnosed with colorectal cancer annually, and more than a third of them will die from it.

The colon cancer cause got a lift from *Today* host Katie Couric, whose husband died in 1998 from colon cancer. Her 2002 on-air colonoscopy on the *Today* show is credited with a 20 percent increase in colonoscopies performed, a spike that researchers dubbed the "Couric Effect."

Couric's on-air advocacy has undoubtedly saved lives, as colon cancer is highly curable when caught early. "You can reduce risk of cancer by about 90 percent by doing regular colonoscopies," says Samuel Meyers, MD, a clinical professor of medicine at Mount Sinai School of Medicine in New York City.

Colon cancer—technically called colorectal cancer—begins with the formation of benign polyps, which can mutate into cancerous tumors. Left untreated, these tumors can penetrate the colon wall and spread.

Colon cancer is predominantly a disease of Westernized societies, and preventable through lifestyle changes. Primitive societies in which people remain physically active and eat diets high in fruits, nuts, and vegetables, low in red meat, and high in fiber simply don't have the colon cancer incidence found in the United States and Europe. Rates of colon cancer in Western Africa, for example, are less than five percent of those in industrialized countries.

What Scientists Know

In a 2004 study, scientists confirmed that diets low in fruits, vegetables and whole grains corresponded to higher rates of colon cancer. These findings echoed a 1997 report from the American Institute for Cancer Research (AICR), which concluded that "[among] the most effective ways of preventing colorectal cancer [is] the consumption of diets high in vegetables."

In addition, specific foods and supplements seem to exert an especially protective effect against colon cancer. High levels of dietary calcium appear to reduce its incidence by as much as 22 percent. The powerful antioxidant selenium is linked to a two-third reduction in polyp recurrence, while studies show that folic acid, which helps prevent DNA damage, can cut colon cancer risk by three quarters. Meyers advises his patients to take all three supplements, as well as to eat generous servings of fruits and vegetables. High blood levels of vitamin D also correlate with lower rates of colon cancer, according to years of research. Diets high in red meat and processed meats such as bologna seem to increase incidence of colon cancer, researchers have reported. In contrast, consumption of fatty fish, which are rich in omega-3 fatty acids, is protective against colon cancer. The AICR recently noted that high intakes of omega-3 fatty acids led to "lower incidences of breast, prostate, and colon cancer than in people who consume less omega-3s."

Studies also show regular use of aspirin is linked to a 20 to 50 percent lower risk of developing colon cancer. And, as it does is with virtually every other chronic disease, exercise plays a role in lowering colon cancer rates. According to the Cancer Research and Prevention Foundation, the evidence is "strong and consistent" that active people have 50 percent lower rates of colon cancer than those who are sedentary.

Confusion abounds about the role of dietary fiber and colon cancer prevention ever since fiber's effectiveness was called into question with studies in 1999 and 2000. However, a 2003 analysis of more 500,000 people in eight countries concluded that people consuming 32 grams of fiber per day were 42 percent less likely to have colon cancer than those consuming the least, or 12 grams a day.

The AICR in 2004 offered an explanation for the confusion: Whole grains, in addition containing fiber, provide powerful antioxidants that likely to protect colon tissue.

Making It Real

As Meyers makes clear, the best way to prevent colon cancer is to detect polyps before they become cancerous.

"It's highly preventable if you have a colonoscopy and you remove the polyp," he says. Many people, however, are squeamish about undergoing a colonoscopy, and put off the important procedure. The primary discomfort associated with it, Meyers says, entails clearing the colon with a laxative the day before, as well as fasting. He says most patients report that the actual procedure isn't as bad as they anticipated.

With the full colonoscopy, the entire rectal and colon area is examined and doctors can remove polyps if spotted during the process. An alternative procedure is called a sigmoidoscopy. This examines the lower third of the colon, where most polyps occur. It's less intrusive than the full colonoscopy but leaves unexamined the rest of the colon, where polyps still occur, albeit with less frequency. For that reason, Meyers discourages its use.

Virtual colonoscopies, a new screening technology, create computer-enhanced X-ray images of the colon, eliminating the invasive step of inserting the flexible tube. However, according to Meyers, most of the older machines in use today miss about 50 percent of the polyps. Some medical major centers have the newest generation of virtual colonoscopy equipment that provides results equivalent to those of standard colonoscopies. And during the next decade, those more accurate machines will likely become more widely available, he says. If you're shopping for a virtual colonoscopy, Meyers advises making sure it offers "multidetector, thin-slice imaging with the ability to tag the stool and eliminate it electronically." Ask your radiologist for details, but realize that without those features, the scan could miss polyps.

To Learn More

For dietary guidelines on lowering colon cancer risk, visit the American Institute for Cancer Research's website at www.aicr.org and click on the "Reducing Your Risk of Colorectal Cancer" icon. Also, visit the American Cancer Society's website at www.cancer.org for information on preventing colon cancer.

CHAPTER 19

Protect Your Prostate

"If a man lives long enough, he'll either die of prostate cancer or with it," goes the wry adage in urology circles. Virtually all men living into their eighties or nineties will have some cancer cells growing in their prostate. Yet many die never realizing they have prostate cancer. This cancer is usually slow-growing, so it can take years for a tumor to grow large enough to detect, and years more for it to spread beyond the prostate. Because it's often caught early, the five-year survival rate for all prostate cancers is 98 percent, according to the Prostate Cancer Foundation. That's the good news. But it occasionally does turn aggressive and deadly.

It's the leading type of non-skin cancer in men. It annually afflicts 230,000 American men and claims nearly 30,000 lives. Some of the best-known men in America have developed (and survived) prostate cancer, including Colin Powell, John Kerry, Rudy Giuliani, and Arnold Palmer.

It's the classic lifestyle disease. Less than 10 percent of cases are genetic, and rates vary sharply between cultures. The evidence "clearly demonstrates there is a relationship between prostate cancer and lifestyle," says Peter Carroll, MD, the head of the urology department at University of California, San Francisco.

What Scientists Know

The prostate, a walnut-sized gland below a man's bladder, surrounds the urethra. The gland produces fluid to mix with semen, pumps semen into the urethra during orgasm, and regulates urine flow. Scientists have known for years that men who regularly consume red meat have a greater probability of developing prostate cancer. In contrast, diets high in seafood (particularly salmon, with its health-boosting omega-3 fatty acids), whole grains, and vegetables reduce prostate cancer risk by as much as 40 percent. Drinking green tea and eating soy also appear to lower risk, according to numerous studies. These lifestyle differences likely explain why Asian men suffer fewer and milder cases of prostate cancer than men in Western cultures, according to Carroll.

Studies show that lycopene, a powerful antioxidant found in tomato-based products like red sauce and tomato juice, is highly effective in keeping prostate cancer at bay. The largest study to date on lycopenes found consuming 2 to 4 servings a week was associated with a

35 percent drop in prostate cancer diagnoses. One remarkable study of men awaiting prostate cancer surgery found that of 12 men given lycopene supplements, tumors shrank in 9 of them, and their cancers became less virulent while their PSA levels declined.

When researchers investigated the ability of the mineral selenium to prevent skin cancer, they came up empty-handed. But to their amazement, they discovered that men taking selenium supplements had a whopping 62 percent reduction in their rate of prostate cancer.

Vitamin E also shows promise in the battle against prostate cancer. The National Institutes of Health is now funding a study with 32,000 men to investigate if vitamin E and selenium will work synergistically to prevent it.

Low levels of vitamin D are correlated with significantly higher rates of prostate cancer. Vitamin D encourages normal cells to remain cancer free and cancer cells to self-destruct. It's also being tested as a possible treatment for prostate cancer, Carroll says.

Wine lovers will be cheered to learn that resveratrol, a phytochemical in red wine, particularly in pinot noir, shows promise in reducing prostate cancer rates.

Those who exercise regularly are also less likely to develop prostate cancer, partly because exercise keeps weight off. In two studies involving more than 800,000 men, the American Cancer Society found a 27 percent increase in prostate cancer deaths in obese men.

Making It Real

If you want a simple formula for preventing prostate cancer, just add some Asian influence to your diet. Cut back on meals with red meat to once or twice a week, and cut back on other sources of dietary fat. We get too much in our culture.

If you're not already a tea drinker, it's a healthful, not to mention pleasurable, habit to adopt. Countless studies show a connection between regular consumption of tea—both black and green—and prostate health.

Like those in Asian cultures, make seafood a regular part of your diet, at least two to three times a week. Select fish high in omega-3 fatty acids, if available. Periodically substitute soy-based foods for meat. If the idea of eating soy leaves you cold, consider using soy milk on cereal, or drinking it mixed with regular milk. It tastes good, and can easily provide you with the 25 to 40 gram intake recommended daily by the Prostate Cancer Foundation.

Going beyond the Asian influence, stock your cupboard with more tomato-based products, such as red sauce and tomato juice, and include them in your diet at least 5 to 7 times a week.

Supplement with 200 mcg daily of yeast-based selenium. Whole grains, wheat germ, and nuts, particularly Brazil nuts, are rich food sources of selenium. Add to that 400 IUs of vitamin E. Also take at least 1000 IUs of vitamin D, or get several minutes of sun about three times a week during the sunny seasons.

Fill your plate with at least 3 to 5 serving a day of vegetables, especially the anti-cancer workhorses in the cruciferous family, like broccoli, cabbage, cauliflower, and brussels sprouts. All are linked to dramatic drops in prostate cancer risk. And fit in at least 2 to 4 servings of fruit per day. According to Carroll, "these dietary changes and these specific supplements are very reasonable" measures to reduce prostate cancer risk.

And here's final bit of good news: an active sex life lowers your risk, according to a study of 30,000 health care professionals.

To Learn More

Visit the Prostate Cancer Foundation's website at www.prostatecancerfoundation.org or the National Cancer Institute's site at http://cancer.gov.

CHAPTER 20

Rise and Dine

"Never work before breakfast; if you have to work before breakfast, eat your breakfast first," wrote Josh Billings, a 19th century humorist. Breakfast, it appears, was high on Mr. Billings's list of priorities in life.

As it should be. The humble meal of breakfast may set the tone not only for the rest of your day, but the quality of your life, according studies on the morning meal's influence on weight, mood, work performance and health.

A good breakfast can reduce the risk of heart disease, diabetes and cancer, while keeping your weight under control. It improves your mood and increases alertness. Yet roughly one-quarter of Americans start their day without the powerful advantage of a good breakfast, according to a federal survey, and numerous studies indicate their performance at work or school suffers as a result.

When you wake in the morning, your blood sugar levels are low, because your body used some of your readily available stores of fuel to keep functioning overnight. Without a morning meal, that low sugar level can cause fatigue, irritability, poor concentration and poor memory. If you decide to skip breakfast, you'll face a morning meeting, a sales presentation, or an exam doing double duty—with your brain struggling to do its best while your body works to convert stored carbohydrates, fat, and proteins into energy. Not exactly a state conducive to peak performance.

Breakfast also provides an ideal opportunity for loading up on high-fiber grains, antioxidant-rich fruits, and cereals fortified with B-vitamins. It's also a chance to get important vitamins and minerals like C, D, and calcium.

What Scientists Know

A common reason people skip breakfast is to lose weight. But the calories saved are frequently offset by binging later on nutritionally poor food, studies show. Skipping breakfast can cause dysregulation of appetite, which makes you unable to tell when you're full, thus leading to the consumption of super-sized meals.

It's actually breakfast eaters, many studies show, that remain the thinnest. A recent University of California, Berkeley analysis of the eating habits of 16,000 Americans found that those eating breakfast had the lowest body mass index, a measurement of body fat, compared with breakfast skippers. People eating cereals, either hot or ready-to-eat, had the lowest body fat. That may be due to the high fiber content of many cereals, which promotes a feeling of satiety, the study authors state.

One study even found that skipping breakfast is also as much of a risk factor for heart disease as smoking or not exercising. Compared to those who didn't eat in the morning, those regularly eating breakfast had lower cholesterol levels. Other researchers found morning cereal eaters had lower levels of the stress hormone cortisol, which can damage the heart and impair cognition. One food in particular, oatmeal, not only lowered LDL cholesterol, but also improved blood pressure, according to another well-publicized study. In addition, many breakfast foods are fortified with B vitamins, including folic acid, which reduces homocysteine levels, an amino acid that can damage the heart.

A Harvard University study with more than 86,000 participants underscored breakfast's role in cardiovascular health, as those who ate whole grain cereal had the lowest rate of death from heart disease. You can also ward off numerous age-related diseases with a sound breakfast. As one study points out, it's an ideal opportunity to get fiber, whole grains, and fruit—foods rich in nutrients and antioxidants credited with slowing the onset of diseases like heart disease and many cancers—all in one bowl.

As the country copes with an alarming rise in Type 2 diabetes rates, breakfast eaters can take comfort knowing that a morning meal helps avoid this preventable disease. Starting the day with a good breakfast that combines high fiber, complex carbohydrates, and moderate levels of protein stabilizes blood sugar levels, a key step for avoiding diabetes. And by avoiding obesity with regular breakfast eating, you'll eliminate the principal risk factor for the disease.

Children perform far better in school, academically and emotionally, when well-fed in the morning, as scores of studies have found. It gives the same mental and emotional edge to adults.

Perhaps because of its influence in preventing so many of the ailments associated with aging, a study of Georgia centenarians reported that among the many traits these elders had in common, one of them was regularly eating breakfast.

Making It Real

In addition to a misguided attempt to lose weight, frantic morning schedules are another reason people skip breakfast. And much of the food people eat on the go, like pastries or fast-food breakfast sandwiches, promote weight gain, says Coralie J.P. Brown, one of the coauthors of the UC Berkeley study. "When people grab food on the run, it's usually higher in fat and simple sugars," she says.

With a little planning, you can easily devise meals-to-go that are nutritionally sound. High-protein fruit smoothies made the night before, or frozen in batches and thawed briefly in a microwave, are an ideal meal to sip in the car. You can make low-calorie breakfast sandwiches ahead of time, like a poached egg on whole wheat bread.

Some people say they can hardly stand the idea of eating in the morning. If those cases, nutritionists urge people to consume something, even if it's a half a glass of orange juice, and then bring healthful, portable food for a mid-morning snack. Try it for a week, nutritionists say, and the difference is noticeable.

For an ideal breakfast, enjoy a bowl of high-fiber cereal with raisins and nuts, or fresh fruit, and top that off with wheat germ. Add lowfat or nonfat milk, or soy milk, and you have a low-calorie, nutritionally dense meal. Also, check the labels on cereal before you buy it, and look for the highest fiber and lowest sugar content.

To Learn More

To learn more about healthy eating habits, visit the website of the American Dietetic Association at www.eatright.org.

CHAPTER 21

Gain the Upper Hand on Breast Cancer

At first glance, the statistics are scary: Roughly 11 percent of women develop breast cancer, about one in every nine women. Breast cancer is the second leading cause of cancer death in women, claiming 40,000 lives annually. But if you look closer, the picture—while very serious—isn't as quite grim as it first appears.

Consider the highly publicized breast cancer fact—that one in every nine women will develop it. While technically correct, that statistic applies over a lifetime to women who reach age 90. When you're 30 years old, your risk is 1 in 5,900 per year; by age 80, it climbs to 1 in 290 per year.

With this confusing stew of statistics, many women overestimate their real risk and suffer needless angst. "Women believe that 40 percent of all deaths are associated with breast cancer, when the correct figure is closer to 4 percent," reports the *Journal of the National Cancer Institute*.

In contrast, nearly 500,000 women die annually from cardiovascular disease, 12 times the number of breast cancer deaths. "I think women are a little too afraid of breast cancer, especially younger women," says Susan Love, MD, a surgeon and well-known author of the bestselling *Dr. Susan Love's Breast Book*. Recovery rates are also improving, thanks to early diagnosis and better treatments. The American Cancer Society states that 97 percent of cases are curable when caught at the local stage.

Certainly concern is merited. Unlike conditions like heart disease, osteoporosis or diabetes, it's not so clear how to prevent breast cancer. "These other ones have reasonable paths of prevention and breast cancer really doesn't," says Love. "I think that makes it scarier." But we're not completely in the dark. Lifestyle changes do make a difference.

What Scientists Know

About ten percent of breast cancers arise from genetic causes. The rest are from "environmental causes" over which you have more control, like food, alcohol, exercise, stress, and obesity.

Exercise is solidly linked to breast cancer protection. Researchers found that moderate exercise—like a brisk 30-minute walk five times a week—reduced the risk by 20 percent. Physical activity helps keep body fat off, offering one explanation for exercise's protective effect. Body fat promotes formation of the hormone estrogen, which plays a role in tumor development. Underscoring that point, excess weight is strongly associated with increased breast cancer risk.

One of the best methods to stay cancer-free is eating fruits and vegetables as a daily habit. They're packed with prevention, and studies show that diets high in fruits and vegetables can provide at least a 20 percent reduction in mortality risk from breast cancer.

A 2004 study reported that women taking aspirin daily had a 28 percent decline in the most common type of breast cancer. Even women taking it once a week had a 20 percent decline. Researchers believe aspirin may block estrogen formation.

You'll likely hear more about vitamin D and cancer prevention, including cancer of the breast. Scientists have learned that vitamin D can coax precancerous cells back to normal and can trigger the death of cancerous cells.

Folic acid is another powerful dietary supplement in the anti-breast-cancer arsenal. Studies show women regularly taking it have lower rates of breast cancer.

Alcohol consumption raises the risk of breast cancer. Researchers from Harvard University calculated that women who have one drink a day increase their lifetime odds by 10 percent; add another drink and the risk goes to 20 percent. Alcohol, they believe, does its damage by stimulating estrogen production.

Researchers think diet provides one explanation for

why women in Asian countries have dramatically lower breast cancer rates than other developed countries. Tea, usually part of the daily ritual, is rich in phytochemicals, which studies suggest protect against breast cancer. Soy is also a dietary staple, and contains isoflavones thought to lower the risk. Fish is another fixture in the Asian diet, providing a steady source of omega-3 fatty acid, which is linked to lower breast cancer rates. Asian women also eat less red meat and other sources of saturated fat. While research is inconclusive about its effect on breast cancer rates, there's no question that diets high saturated fat cause other health problems.

Making It Real

What's the first step you should take to prevent breast cancer? Well, it's just that—take a step and keep walking, for about 30 minutes a day and ideally at least five days a week. Numerous types of activity offer the same benefit, like biking, swimming, or running. However, a walking habit is one of the easiest to adopt.

Eat generous amounts of fruits and vegetables, and you'll also protect yourself against diseases ranging from heart disease to diabetes. And limit your consumption of red meat, butter, and other sources of saturated fats. If you drink, go easy on alcohol consumption. It's an easy way to reduce your risk. Be sure to take 800 mcg of folic acid daily. It's especially important if you drink, as studies indicate it can counteract the increased risk linked to drinking. Add soy-based foods to your diet. There are some delicious prepared ones on the market, if regular tofu isn't appealing to you. Make sure to eat food high in omega-3 fatty acids—like salmon, trout or flax seed—at least twice a week.

While it's too soon to recommend aspirin to lower breast cancer risk, women considered at high risk should talk with their doctors about the tradeoffs of starting now, as aspirin offers other health benefits.

With convincing evidence accumulating that vitamin D offers cancer protection, some scientists believe it's good medicine to get regular, but brief, sun exposure. (Sun creates vitamin D when rays hit your skin.) Or you can rely on vitamin D supplements. Experts in vitamin D research go beyond the federal guidelines and recommend up to 1000 IUs a day.

To Learn More

For an understanding of breast cancer risks and prevention strategies, visit www.breastcancer.org and the Centers for Disease Control and Prevention website on breast cancer at www.cdc.gov/cancer/nbccedp.

CHAPTER 22

Detect Breast Cancer Early

Breast cancer mortality rates have declined by more than 20 percent since 1989, a fortunate trend credited to improved treatment and to an increased usage of mammograms. By peering inside the body with imaging tools like mammography to look for tumors—a process called screening—women have a better chance of detecting cancer before it spreads. When breast cancer is found early at the localized stage, 97 percent of women will survive it.

Mammograms are the best tool available for breast cancer screenings, although they're far from ideal. Health agencies are pushing for better technologies, which are emerging but still have drawbacks. The prestigious Institute of Medicine, which in a 2004 report praised mammography's role in reducing breast cancer mortality, also notes that it can miss tumors and flags many benign lumps that nonetheless require women to endure a tissue biopsy to rule out cancer.

Another drawback to mammography is its use of radiation, of which the Food and Drug Administration states there's no safe exposure level. Health professionals, however, say mammography machines emit very low levels, and the benefits outweigh the risks.

Mammography is also less accurate in women under age 50, because their breasts are denser and X-rays don't penetrate as well.

Susan Love, MD, a surgeon and author of a bestselling book on breast health, also advocates aggressive research on ductal lavage, which can detect cells in milk ducts—where all breast cancers start—that are on the verge of becoming cancerous. When found at this stage, there's virtually a 100 percent recovery rate.

What Scientists Know

Despite its litany of drawbacks, breast cancer experts— Love among them—are in agreement that women should get regular mammograms while other technologies are under development. It still certainly saves lives.

Ultrasound screening is one of the more promising new techniques for increasing breast tumor detection rates, as an augment to mammograms. One study found that mammography only detected tumors in 48 percent of women with very dense breasts. When ultrasound was also used, 94 percent of the cancers were found. A 2004 study reports that ultrasound screening is superior to mammograms for detecting invasive breast cancers.

Digital mammography, approved by the FDA in 2000, is another recent advance. With this technique, the X-ray images are stored digitally, instead of on film. This allows a radiologist to zoom in on a suspicious image, and the computer also flags unusual areas, providing a double read. The digital image can easily be shared with other health professionals.

In one study, digital mammography detected nearly 20 percent more breast cancers than mammography, although other studies found no difference between the two. Love, for one, isn't entirely sold on digital mammography. "If anything, it's not as sensitive as regular mammography." She suggests that there may be a trade off between the double read and the ease of sharing the image with other health professionals.

Magnetic resonance imaging, or MRI, generates detailed images without using radiation. A recent study found that MRI was significantly more sensitive than mammograms in detecting tumors in women with a genetic risk for breast cancer.

With ductal lavage, the nipple is anesthetized and a hair-thin catheter thread in. It then sucks out cells from the milk duct, which are then examined for abnormalities. Love believes ductal lavage may eventually be used routinely to catch breast cancer in its incipient—and curable—stage. But the technique for assessing abnormal cells is currently too unreliable for widespread use.

Conventional clinical breast exams, in which a health professional feels breasts for lumps and other abnormalities, are strongly advised by the American Cancer Society to augment mammograms.

Enthusiasm is waning for breast self-exams. Even the American Cancer Society says women can consider it optional. The reasons? The process often makes women anxious and studies show it's not effective in catching cancers early.

Making It Real

Major health care organizations recommend that women age 40 and older get annual mammograms.

But brace yourself for the confusing controversy of whether women in their forties should get a regular mammogram, exposing themselves to radiation and a possible biopsy. Four out of five times, lumps detected by mammography are benign.

The American Cancer Society expresses confidence that screening should start in a woman's forties. As stated on their website: "Recent evidence has confirmed that mammograms offer substantial benefit for women in their forties."

The federal government, however, isn't as firm in that recommendation. The U.S. Preventive Services Task Force stated that debate over the benefit of mammography in that age group "makes it difficult to determine the incremental benefit of beginning screening at age 40 rather than at age 50."

Love says she doesn't recommend women in their forties get an annual mammogram, in part because of the X-ray exposure and in part because of the perplexing "mammogram paradox." The paradox refers studies finding that women in their forties getting a mammogram actually have higher mortality rates from breast cancer than women in their forties not getting them. Other studies, however, do show a survival benefit.

Still, many people know of women in their forties whose cancer was caught early, thanks to a mammogram. So women have to navigate this controversial issue using their own informed judgment. But women over age 50 should have a mammogram every 12 to 16 months, the task force recommended.

Women in their twenties and thirties should also have a clinical breast exam at least once every 3 years. At age 40 and beyond, women should have an annual clinical breast exam.

To Learn More

For more information, visit the National Cancer Institute's website at www.nci.nih.gov. Type in "mammograms" in the Search box.

CHAPTER 23

Stay Young with Strong Legs

For a want of the nail, a shoe was lost,
For want of the shoe, the horse was lost,
For the want of the horse, the rider was lost,
For the want of the rider….

You know the rest. So how does Benjamin Franklin's adage connect to strong legs? Simple—let your leg strength decline over time, and you'll set in motion a cascade of events that could lead to disability or even premature death. With weakened legs, you'll first avoid activities that require exertion, like long walks or biking. Then, getting out of a chair or ascending a flight of stairs becomes a challenge. As muscle further deteriorates, you may need a cane or a walker to safely get around.

When you do stand without assistance, like getting out of the shower, you're vulnerable to a hip-breaking fall, because your balance isn't so good and you don't have the reflexes to break a fall. If you're unfortunate enough to break a hip, you'll end up in the hospital. Because of post-surgical complications that often arise, 25 percent of older people with hip fractures don't survive the first year after their fall. If you do survive, you'll feel very depressed and old before your time.

This specter of shuffling around with a cane or navigating in a wheelchair due to the loss of leg strength is usually preventable, says Irwin Rosenberg, MD, a senior scientist with the Human Nutrition Research Center on Aging at Tufts University. Rosenberg first named the condition of age-related muscle loss, using the Greek word "sarcopenia," which means "vanishing flesh."

"There is in fact an antidote, and that is resistance exercise," he says. "Some decline in strength and muscle mass is associated with aging. But it need not lead to disability."

What Scientists Know

So why the focus on leg strength? While overall body strength is vital for maintaining independence, it's particularly true for the lower limbs. Strong legs, studies show, are your insurance policy for an active and enjoyable life in your later years.

In fact, strength training may be the preferred exercise the older you get, says Jeffrey Potteiger, PhD, chair of the Department of Physical Education at Miami University in Ohio. "You could make an argument that it's more important for an older adult to maintain strength than to maintain cardiovascular fitness," he says. "At the very least it's equally important." It's also safe, if done in moderation.

Older people who strength train their legs begin to reclaim some of their lost youthful agility. A Tufts University study found that men and women in their eighties and nineties who began resistance training started walking faster, climbing more stairs, and attaining better balance and reflexes; in a few cases the subjects gave up their walkers.

The workout doesn't have to be strenuous. Older men who worked out lightly three times a week showed up to a 22 percent increase in leg muscle mass. Higher intensity programs yield more dramatic results. A group of men, average age 64, who weight trained intensely three times a week experienced as much as a tripling in leg strength.

Fit leg muscles also protect knee joints. With age, thigh muscles weaken from lack of exercise, and more of the mechanical stress of walking, running, and standing transfers to the knee joint. Strong leg muscles help absorb that stress, and prevent the breakdown of cartilage and the onset of osteoarthritis.

Muscles weakened from age and disuse are just as important risk factors for hip fractures in elders as weakened bones, health experts are realizing. The two conditions—sarcopenia and osteoporosis—are two sides of the same coin. (Sarcopenia is also costly, running up $18.5 billion in health care costs in 2000.) A study in the *Journal of the American Medical Association* found that weakened lower limbs and postural instability increased risk of hip fracture, one of the leading reasons that elders end up wheelchair bound. And as anyone who's ever had to use crutches can attest, disability and depression often go hand in hand. Many studies link impaired mobility with moderate to severe depression, which then takes people on a steady decline, as motivation to improve fades.

Making It Real

Leg exercises are often the most neglected part of a workout program, as exercisers focus on developing a buff upper body. Don't ignore your lower body when working out.

Two of the best leg exercises in the gym are pedaling the stationary bike, set at moderate resistance, and using the leg press machine. With the bike, you get aerobic and resistance training in the same workout. Both exercises isolate the thigh muscle for maximum gain, in addition to working other leg muscles.

There are excellent exercises you can perform at home. Climb stairs, and if you're ambitious, do two at a time. Five minutes daily will strengthen legs and provide a mild aerobic workout.

Stand on one leg, moderately bent, for at least 15 seconds. Then alternate with the other leg. This exercise transfers all of your weight onto one leg, giving leg muscles an isometric workout. This also stresses the bones of the leg and hip, helping to maintain bone density. This simple routine also improves balance.

Here's an exercise you can do while seated watching television. Just stand up and sit down 20 times in succession. That's a superb leg strengthener.

For more ideas on leg exercises, pick up a strength training book, visit the Centers for Disease Control and Prevention's website on strength training, listed below, or work with a certified personal trainer. If you're over age 65, or have risk factors for heart disease, visit your physician before starting a strength training program.

Remember to always warm up with a mild aerobic exercise, like walking, before weight training, and to stretch afterward.

To Learn More

Visit the Centers for Disease Control and Prevention's website, which provides a free detailed guide for beginning a strength training program:

www.cdc.gov/nccdphp/dnpa/physical/growing_stronger

CHAPTER 24

Find Your Place in the Sun

About 25 years ago, the strange distribution of colon cancer in the United States caught two researchers' attention. The farther north citizens lived, the greater their probability of developing it. Rates were twice as high in the northeast as in the southwest. Later, a NASA scientist found similar patterns for 15 other types of cancer, including that of the breast, prostate, esophagus, and ovaries.

Multiple sclerosis rates also climb the farther people live from the equator, as does the frequency of hypertension. The prescient scientists concluded that a lack of vitamin D explained these unusual disease patterns in the often sun-deprived northern latitudes. Until then, vitamin D, created by the body when sun hits the skin, was widely known only for its role in maintaining bone and teeth health.

No longer. Piles of studies link low vitamin D levels to a range of unrelated diseases, from cancers and diabetes to heart disease and rheumatoid arthritis. "Almost every tissue and organ in the body recognizes activated vitamin

D," says Michael Holick, MD, PhD, a researcher at Boston University Medical Center and one the nation's authorities on vitamin D. This means that, for reasons under investigation, a number of metabolic processes depend on vitamin D to proceed normally.

At the same time, the U.S. population is shockingly deficient in the vitamin. "I estimate 30 percent to 50 percent of the U.S. population is either chronically or seasonally deficient in vitamin D," Holick says.

This shortfall alone may cause 30,000 cancer deaths annually in the United States, according to one estimate.

Holick says that lifestyles adopted over the past 50 years, which keep people indoors more often, as well as the "scare tactics" used by professional dermatology associations about sun exposure and skin cancer, largely explains this endemic vitamin D deficiency.

What Scientists Know

We all become vitamin D factories when the sun's UVB rays strike our skin. Vitamin D is stored in fat, enabling humans to generate it during the sunny months and pull from reserves in the winter. Holick says that north of about 35 degrees latitude, where Atlanta, Georgia lies, little or no UVB rays reach the ground during the winter, as they're absorbed in the atmosphere due to the angle of the sun. Thus, it can be difficult to get all the UVB rays you need, especially during the winter.

Vitamin D is essential for capturing and employing the calcium we ingest. Without it, the small intestine only absorbs about 15 percent of consumed calcium, with the rest passing unused. Vitamin D also helps lay down calcium onto bones and teeth to harden them.

In one analysis, researchers found that older women taking at least 400 IUs daily of vitamin D had 20 percent fewer injuries from falls, particularly hip fractures, compared with those deficient in the vitamin.

But it has a far more dynamic role than simply maintaining healthy bones and teeth.

Vitamin D coaxes cells on the verge of becoming cancerous back to normal and away from runaway replication, a hallmark of cancer. It also induces the death of cancerous cells. Cancers of the breast, ovary, prostate and colon diminish after exposure to vitamin D in laboratory experiments. A 2005 study from Harvard University concludes that adequate levels of vitamin D would reduce the rates for all cancers by at least 30 percent.

An analysis of more than 5,000 women found that those living in sunny climates had between a 25 percent to 65 percent drop in breast cancer risk.

Prostate cancer cells have vitamin D receptors, Stanford University researchers report, and when vitamin D latches on, it reduces cancer cell proliferation.

The "sunshine vitamin" helps keep the immune system from turning on the body, the cause of autoimmune diseases like multiple sclerosis, rheumatoid arthritis, and

Type 1 diabetes. "Vitamin D is one of the most potent regulators of the immune system," says Holick.

Cardiovascular health is also supported by vitamin D, probably by inhibiting renin production, an enzyme that raises blood pressure. It also helps prevent cardiomyopathy, or "enlarged heart," which can lead to heart failure.

Holick is certain that osteomalacia, a condition in which bones become softened by insufficient vitamin D, is frequently misdiagnosed as a perplexing syndrome called fibromyalgia. Osteomalacia causes muscle pain and weakness, the classic symptoms of fibromyalgia.

Making It Real

Federal guidelines advise people up to age 50 to consume 200 IUs of vitamin D daily; 400 IUs for those ages 51 to 70; and 600 IUs for those 71 and older. But Holick and other experts advise 1,000 IUs a day, through a combination of sun, supplements, and food.

Since vitamin D is stored in fat, don't overdo it with supplements; however, one study concluded that to build up toxic amounts of the vitamin would require consuming at least 40,000 IUs daily for months. There are few adequate food sources of vitamin D aside from fatty fish like salmon or cod. Milk is enriched with vitamin D, although Holick and colleagues found that the actual levels of vitamins the food contained were often lower than stated on the carton. Orange juice and cereal are sometimes supplemented with the vitamin, and Holick says those levels are more reliable.

That leaves sunshine or supplements to fill the gap. The most effective supplement is vitamin D3 or cholecalciferol, a natural version equivalent to vitamin D formed by sun.

Holick, to the dismay of many dermatologists, says people can safely sun to build up vitamin D reserves. He advises measuring the time it takes your skin to turn pink (not burned) in full sun. Then sit in the sun for a quarter of that time, two to three times a week. Those with darker skin need longer exposure. As skin cancers commonly appear on the face and ears, cover those areas and sun your legs and arms. If you remain outside longer, put on sunscreen.

It's a good idea to get your vitamin D level tested. It costs about $100 and may be covered by health insurance. Make sure your doctor tests for the partially active form, 25 hydroxy-vitamin D, a much more reliable measurement than the active form.

To Learn More

Read Dr. Michael Holick's book *The UV Advantage*.

CHAPTER 25

Fight Back with Folic Acid

Folic acid, a vitamin vital to normal cell division, growth, and DNA repair, has finally gotten some respect from the Food and Drug Administration. In 1998, after years of debate, the agency directed manufacturers of enriched grain products like flour, bread, cereal, and pasta to start adding folic acid to their products. It was the first time in more than 50 years that the FDA forced manufacturers to supplement food products to protect the public from the health hazard of nutritional deficiency.

The FDA issued the mandate to ensure that pregnant women consume enough folic acid to prevent certain birth defects, and rates of those abnormalities have since declined 20 percent. However, scientists have long known that folic acid deficiency is also linked to adult diseases. Striking evidence indicates it prevents strokes and heart attacks. In a stunning announcement, federal health officials reported in 2004 that more than 48,000 strokes and heart attacks appear to have been prevented by the folic acid grain supplementation. Other research shows that folic acid significantly lowers the incidence of colon cancer, and may ward off osteoporosis and Alzheimer's disease.

Folic acid is "central to life," says Godfrey Oakley Jr., MD, MPH, a professor of epidemiology at Emory University in Atlanta and a leading advocate for increasing folic acid intake.

While the declines in birth defects and now cardiovascular disease are encouraging, Oakley says much of the U.S. population is still deficient in the versatile vitamin, as the FDA stopped far short of mandating an adequate supplementation level.

What Scientists Know

Folic acid plays a hand in the creation, replication and repair of DNA, while guarding the integrity of your genetic blueprint against potentially cancerous changes. It provides the building blocks needed by rapidly dividing cells, such as those in an embryo. In developing embryos, it protects against birth defects, primarily spina bifida, a neurological deformity in which the spine doesn't fully close, as well as anencephaly and cleft palate. "If you can't make cells, or if you can't make DNA or keep it repaired, your body is in trouble," Oakley says.

Folic acid also maintains proper blood levels of the amino acid homocysteine, a by-product of dietary protein metabolism. Scientists believe optimal folic acid levels protect against heart disease and stroke by lowering levels of homocysteine, which can damage artery walls. While your body needs some homocysteine, excess amounts are now considered an independent risk factor for cardiovascular disease.

Low folic acid levels also contribute to the development of certain cancers, numerous studies suggest. When folic acid levels are low, the risk of an error in DNA replication or repair—and hence cancer—increases. Low folic acid can also trigger critical genes to inappropriately turn on or off, wreaking havoc in the body. Oakley cites the work of Bruce Ames, PhD, a world-renowned scientist from the University of California at Berkeley who believes that folic acid deficiency explains more cancer cases than any other cause. A Harvard University study of more than 88,000 women found that those with a hereditary predisposition for developing colon cancer could sharply reduce that risk by consuming a daily multivitamin containing folic acid. Another study of more than 32,000 women linked high folic acid levels to lower rates of breast cancer, especially in women at higher risk because of alcohol intake. Other research suggests a connection between low folic acid levels and cancers of the esophagus, cervix, lung, and pancreas.

A new crop of studies finds a connection between high homocysteine, low folic acid levels, and the onset of Alzheimer's disease. Low levels are also linked to poor cognition and depression. In addition, researchers believe osteoporosis may be associated with high homocysteine levels, as excess amounts of the amino acid—a by-product of animal protein metabolism—may interfere with normal formation of collagen, a tissue which strengthens bones.

Making It Real

Oakley has a major complaint with the FDA's folic acid supplement regulation—it didn't go nearly far enough. Adults need at least 400 mcg/day to receive all the benefit of folic acid. Despite urging from the U.S. Centers for Disease Control and Prevention for higher supplementation levels, the FDA mandated levels so low that the typical daily consumption of enriched grain products provides only 100 mcg/day.

Folic acid is an unusual vitamin in that people need supplements to get an adequate amount, Oakley says. That's not to dismiss important food sources, such as dark leafy vegetables and citrus fruit. However, the average serving of a fruit or vegetable contains 40 mcg or less of the vitamin. And, as Oakley observed, Americans rarely consume the recommended quantity of fruits and vegetables. "It's more like 20 a day that's needed, and we can't even get to five a day," he says.

Another hurdle is that only about half of the naturally occurring vitamin found in food is absorbed. In contrast, nearly all of the supplemental form makes its way into your system.

Oakley advises everyone to take a multivitamin, as the costs are low, the risks nil, and the upside tremendous. If you purchase a separate folic acid supplement, make sure it's combined with B12, which works in concert with folic acid. Oakley also notes that many cereal manufacturers now fortify a single serving of their product with 400 mcg of folic acid, and "have probably saved lots of people's lives."

Take between 400 mcg and 800 mcg/day. But there's no need to take more, unless your doctor recommends it, for example, to lower your homocysteine level. Oakley says it's virtually impossible to ingest toxic levels the water-soluble vitamin, adding that a case study of someone getting 50,000 mcg/day found no adverse effects. If you're on chemotherapy, talk with your doctor before using folic acid.

To Learn More

Visit the National Council on Folic Acid's website at www.folicacidinfo.org. The nonprofit council is funded by partnership of more than 80 national organizations and government agencies.

CHAPTER 26

Eat Like a Caveman

During the Paleolithic Era, which ended 10,000 years ago with the advent of agriculture, humans moved about in nomadic hunter-gatherer tribes. They ate the food they could trap, kill, pluck from plants or dig from the ground.

Although our primitive ancestors consumed a great deal of meat, it contained far less of the unhealthy saturated fats found in today's grain-fed livestock. While they could not always count on a meal of game animals, plants virtually guaranteed a steady source of sustenance.

Vegetables were in fact a mainstay, providing a large portion of their diet. They picked mounds of leaves, cut armfuls of edible stems and unearthed piles of starchy bulbs. They occasionally gathered grass seeds, but otherwise ate few grains. Our Stone Age ancestors enjoyed meals dense with nutrients, phytochemicals, antioxidants, and fiber.

Today, a cadre of nutritionists insists our bodies genetically evolved to thrive on that balance of primitive fare.

In their view, our modern diets are nutritional disasters, in which refined carbohydrates and meats high in saturated fat dominate our plates and vegetables are often just a soggy side dish.

While their views occupy the fringe in nutrition circles, virtually every dietary expert agrees these "Paleo enthusiasts" have a point: Early humans ate a better variety and greater quantity of plant-based foods than we do today. That may explain why populations today that eat generous amounts of vegetables suffer far fewer chronic diseases than groups that don't.

What Scientists Know

For years, we've known that vegetables contain important vitamins, minerals, and fiber. But what's new is the growing appreciation of the nutritional value of the more than 4,000 phytochemicals and antioxidants that plant-based foods provide.

Plants evolved these chemicals in part to protect themselves from threats posed by microbes, insects, genetic mutations, and excess cold, heat, or drought. And those same chemicals that protect plants from harm often do the same for humans.

Studies of the eating habits of populations worldwide alerted scientists to the protective effects of a diet high in plant-based foods. In Italy, researchers found that a group of healthy centenarians ate twice as many vegetables as their younger counterparts. Seventh Day Adventists, who usually follow a vegetarian diet or eat meat sparingly, have been intensely studied and results show they have lower rates of cardiovascular disease, diabetes, hypertension, arthritis, dementia, obesity, and several types of cancer. Recent research concludes that a vegetarian diet is as effective as statin drugs in lowering cholesterol levels. And eating vegetables can give your skin a more youthful appearance, according to another study.

While all vegetables provide nutrients and beneficial phytochemicals, some are standouts. Members of the Cruciferae family—like broccoli, cabbage, brussels sprouts, and cauliflower—contain phytochemicals in abundance. Of great interest is a phytochemical called sulforaphane. Studies show it may thwart the growth of some cancers, including that of the prostate and breast. Sprouts of broccoli, cauliflower, alfalfa, radish, and clover contain even more concentrated amounts of this beneficial plant compound. These vegetables also contain several other phytochemicals known for their cancer-fighting properties.

Bell peppers are loaded with fiber and nutrients like vitamins B6 and C. Red and orange varieties are also great sources of carotenoids. Spinach is rich in riboflavin, vitamin B6, magnesium, and folate, as well as carotenoids. The ever-popular tomato is another nutritional king. Technically a fruit, it provides fiber, vitamin C, some B vitamins, iron, and potassium, as well as an important carotenoid found in few other vegetables called lycopene.

Lycopene is particularly abundant in tomato reductions like tomato sauce, paste and juice. Persuasive studies link diets high in lycopene to reduced rates of prostate cancer and, more recently, cardiovascular disease. Because carotenoids are fat soluble, meaning they mix with oil but not water, they're best absorbed when prepared or eaten with a fat like olive oil.

The lowly bean, the "poor man's meat," is rightfully gaining respect. Beans, such as the familiar kidney and pinto beans, are rich in antioxidants, B vitamins and minerals like potassium. They're high in protein and—unlike meat—come without the baggage of saturated fats. They also pack ample amounts of soluble and insoluble fiber which can help clear out cholesterol and regulate your digestive tract.

Sweet potatoes are another standout. They contain vitamins B6 and C, iron, potassium, a rich store of carotenoids, and a surprisingly generous amount of vitamin E.

Making It Real

If you enjoy indulging in a hefty meal, you can load up on vegetables guilt-free. Learn to prepare flavorful recipes, like a low calorie sauce over broccoli, a savory vegetable soup, or spicy cauliflower, and you could find yourself getting hooked. Filling up on vegetables will also leave you satiated and less drawn to high calorie, nutritionally poor foods.

Pick richly-colored vegetables to get a bounty of nutrients. It's generally best to consume fresh vegetables, as most of the nutrients are intact. There are exceptions, however. Fresh vegetables lose more nutrients the longer they are stored. In contrast, vegetables processed for freezing are often flash-frozen shortly after harvest, locking in their nutrients. Canned vegetables are OK, but not optimal. Many of their nutrients, like vitamins B and C, are lost in the heat of processing. Canned vegetables also contain high sodium levels.

While potatoes are the most popular vegetable in the United States, eat white-fleshed potatoes sparingly. They spike blood glucose levels, and are short on many nutrients in comparison to other vegetables. And they're frequently deep-fried, which virtually negates any nutritional benefits they offer.

To Learn More

Visit the U.S. Centers for Disease Control and Prevention's "5 A Day" website at www.cdc.gov/nccdphp/dnpa/5aday. The site offers ideas for incorporating at least five servings of vegetables and fruits into your diet, and provides easy, low-calorie recipes.

CHAPTER 27

Forage for Fruits

The Paleolithic hunter-gatherers who roamed grasslands in search of game and edible plants also included an abundance of wild fruits in their regular fare. They enjoyed a wide variety—blueberries, strawberries, and gooseberries, stone fruits like apricots and plums, or apples, pears, pomegranates, and grapes. This colorful and tasty bounty not only satisfied the ancient sweet tooth, but provided a rich source of vitamins, minerals, and antioxidants that complemented those found in vegetables.

Fruits generally surpass vegetables in their levels of antioxidants, those free radical scavengers that protect cellular components, including DNA, from damage by charged-up oxygen molecules. Blueberries, for example, deliver twice the amount of antioxidants as spinach, and three times that of broccoli. Many nutritionists believe that, thanks to evolution, we're now hard-wired to need a steady supply of antioxidants and other phytochemicals for optimal health. Historical studies, as well as research on indigenous cultures intact today, show people adhering to diets high in plant foods are largely free of the degenerative diseases common in modern societies.

Fruits are also rich in soluble fiber, the kind that clears out cholesterol and stabilizes blood sugars. Like vegetables, they contain no cholesterol and, with rare exception, contain no fat. How many foods can boast those virtues?

What Scientists Know

The oxygen you breathe fires virtually all your body's functions, down to the individual cell. But once inside, some oxygen molecules lose or gain electrons and transform themselves into unstable free radicals. These reactive molecules then rampage through your body, seeking to steal an electron or dump one off on a stable molecule, in turn converting that one into a new free radical. It's this cascade of molecular events that causes iron to rust, fats to turn rancid, and you to age prematurely.

In humans, studies show free radicals can damage cells in the heart, brain, organs, artery walls, eyes, and skin. They can infiltrate into DNA, damaging genetic material and potentially triggering cancerous mutations. And many scientists believe it's the engine behind the process of aging and ultimately death.

But we're not defenseless against this cellular assault. In fact, nature provided us with foods, in particular fruits and vegetables, can mount a masterful counteroffensive.

These foods deploy the familiar antioxidant vitamins, like vitamins E and C, as well as an army of plant compounds called phytochemicals. Scientists believe there are thousands of different phytochemicals in plant-based foods, although we've only closely studied a few hundred. Many of these phytochemicals also serve as antioxidants that neutralize free radicals or repair the cellular damage caused by them.

Fruits can help you live longer. A 26-year study of Swedish men found that those who ate the most fruit had lower death rates from cardiovascular disease. Another study showed that rates of dementia decreased in participants eating the highest levels of fruit. One remarkable animal study reported that rats genetically predisposed to Alzheimer's disease but also fed blueberry supplements didn't develop the disease, while genetically identical rats deprived of the supplement did. The researchers concluded that it may be possible with diet to overcome even a hereditary vulnerability to Alzheimer's. A recent animal study with blueberry phytochemicals found the plant compounds lowered cholesterol better than a prescription drug.

Fruits like apples, oranges, berries, apricots and prunes, which are rich in soluble fiber, can lower total and LDL cholesterol. An interesting study on the soluble fibers in guava juice concluded that the fibers not only reduced total cholesterol and triglycerides, but led to a "substantial reduction" in blood pressure. All are risk factors for cardiovascular disease.

Cultivating a taste for fruit may also preserve your eyesight later in life, according to a 2004 study with more than 117,000 participants. Scientists reported that those eating at least three pieces of fruit daily had a 36 percent lower risk of developing age-related macular degeneration—the leading cause of vision loss in Americans aged 60 and older—compared with those who ate fewer than 1.5 pieces daily.

Fruit is also rich in potassium, and researchers have recently found a link between high intake of this mineral and lowered stroke incidence. Daily consumption of just one banana, which is high in potassium, significantly reduced stroke risk, one study found.

And we can't overlook fruits' original claim to fame—their abundance of essential vitamins like A and C, and minerals such as magnesium.

Making It Real

Like vegetables, the fruit family also has its standouts. Blueberries are remarkably rich in antioxidants, with a half cup providing at least 10 times the amount of antioxidants as a medium-sized apple. And prunes provide more than twice the amount as a serving of blueberries.

Other fruits high in antioxidants, in descending order, are raisins, blackberries, strawberries, raspberries, plums, oranges, red grapes, and cherries, according to the U.S. Department of Agriculture. But all fruits contain antioxidants, so feel free to regularly enjoy your favorites, rather than only concentrating on the antioxidant superstars.

Nutritionists repeatedly advise consumers to eat whole fruit, rather than rely on supplements. For one reason, supplement levels are wildly unreliable, according to a study by the USDA. More importantly, scientists are certain that the myriad of phytochemicals in fruit work synergistically with one another. They also know there are many more phytochemicals awaiting discovery, some of which will likely prove valuable to human health.

At minimum, health experts advise eating four pieces of fruit a day. Part of that can be in the form of juice, although the tradeoff is a loss of valuable fiber and blood sugar stability. Fruit smoothies, which retain the fiber, are an easy way to pack at least two fruit servings into one meal. Frozen fruit is nutritionally equivalent to fresh fruit. Canned fruit is an acceptable alternative, although some nutrients and phytochemicals are lost during processing. They're also often canned in sugary syrup.

To Learn More

Visit the Harvard University's School of Public Health website at www.hsph.harvard.edu/nutritionsource and click on the "Fruit & Vegetables" icon.

CHAPTER 28

Get into Grains

A bowl of Cocoa Puffs, the top of a hamburger bun, a slice of whole wheat bread, and a donut have one thing in common—they're all considered a serving of grain by the U.S. Department of Agriculture's Dietary Guidelines for Americans.

And that's not only wrong, many prominent nutritionists say, but a disservice to the public. A donut or a serving of sugary cereal are more akin to a dessert than a healthful serving of grains, and American's are paying for the muddled classification with their waistlines and their health.

Walter Willett, MD, the chair of the nutrition department at Harvard's School of Public Health and influential voice in nutrition policy who has long advocated for changes to the USDA's food pyramid, scored a victory in 2005 when the federal agency updated its advice on grain consumption. The agency now advises that people consume at least three servings a day of whole grain foods, whereas previously it made no distinction between whole and refined grain foods. "The new guidelines do represent important progress compared to the current food guide pyramid," Willett states in a *San Francisco Chronicle* article. But the new pyramid still gives its blessings for the consumption of too many refined starches, Willett says.

However, the Grocery Manufacturers of America, one of many trade groups influencing the pyramid's content, insists it's important to keep refined grain-based products in the mix. The federal government, it points out, requires food manufacturers to enrich refined grain products with folic acid, niacin, thiamin, riboflavin, and iron.

Here's why the irrefutable evidence of Willett and others has swayed the agency entrusted with advising Americans on what to eat for optimal health.

What Scientists Know

Grains are seeds harvested from plants in the grass family, like wheat, corn and oats. A thin, nutritious layer called bran surrounds the carbohydrate-rich endosperm, which encapsulates the inner germ layer. Together, the bran and germ layer contain most of the grain's nutrients, such as folate, B vitamins, vitamin E, and the minerals potassium, magnesium, selenium, copper, and zinc. Grains are also sources of phytoestrogens, which inhibit hormones like estrogen in promoting cancers. In addition, whole grains are rich in soluble fibers that stabilize blood sugar levels and lower total and LDL cholesterol levels.

But to improve the appearance and shelf life of grain-based foods, manufacturers strip away the bran and germ, leaving only the thick starchy middle layer. Most cereals and baked goods are made from these processed grains. Lacking the fiber-rich and nutritious bran and germ, the processed grain digests quickly, spiking blood sugar and insulin levels. If this happens too often, the risk of developing diabetes increases.

Aside from the nutrients that manufacturers must add by law, processed grains are essentially devoid of vitamins, minerals and phytoestrogens. Not surprisingly, large studies have found that people eating three servings a day of whole-grain foods were up to one-third less likely to develop Type 2 diabetes than those rarely or never eating whole grains. The soluble fibers in whole grains likely explain the protective effect.

Numerous studies decisively show that whole grain foods protect your heart. Diets high in these grains tend to decrease levels of LDL, increase HDL and lower triglyceride levels. They are also linked to lower blood pressure and homocysteine levels. A recent study reports that participants consuming the highest levels of whole grains had a 29 percent lower risk of developing cardiovascular disease. The researchers concluded that "whole grain foods may be one of the healthiest choices individuals can make to lower the risk for atherosclerotic cardiovascular disease." In the face of this evidence, the Food and Drug Administration now permits labels on whole grain foods to state that whole grains protect against heart disease and some cancers.

A convincing case has also been made for the protective effect of whole grains against cancer. An analysis of 40 studies linked high intakes of whole grains to a 34 percent risk reduction in several cancers. The most consistent connection involved cancers of the gastrointestinal tract—the mouth, throat, stomach, colon and rectum. The fiber in whole grains also helps prevent constipation and painful diverticulitis.

Making It Real

It doesn't take copious amounts of whole grains to enjoy these health benefits—only two to three servings a day, according to studies. But most Americans, despite high consumption of grain-based products, get less than one serving per day of whole grains. This is due in part to consumers' resistance to the dark color, richer flavor and coarser texture of these foods. And, as Willett points out in his book, whole grain foods may be a little harder to find and take longer to cook.

You will find whole grains foods can be delicious, once you drop the refined flour habit. If local stores don't carry items like whole wheat pastas and nutritious grains, such as amaranth, quinoa, or buckwheat, online retailers will.

It's easy to include more whole grains in your diet. For example, have a whole grain cereal for breakfast, two slices of whole grain bread at lunch, and serve whole grain pasta for dinner.

Labels can be misleading. Make sure they say "whole wheat flour," not just "wheat flour." The latter is in fact refined, stripped of its bran and germ.

One note: Refined grain products are also enriched with folic acid, niacin, thiamin, riboflavin, and iron. Whole grains, however, aren't generally fortified, and the U.S. population is often deficient in these nutrients. Be sure to get sufficient amounts through other food sources or supplements.

Finally, ignore the USDA recommendation of six to eleven daily grain servings. Unless they are intact grains, they are largely empty calories. Instead, focus on getting three to four whole grain servings daily, substituting fruits and vegetables for those other recommended grain servings.

To Learn More

Visit the Harvard School of Public Health website at www.hsph.harvard.edu/nutritionsource and select the "Carbohydrates" icon.

To view the federal government's "Dietary Guidelines for Americans," visit www.healthierus.gov/dietaryguidelines.

CHAPTER 29

Rough It

Fiber provides negligible calories, but it fills you up. It's not a vitamin, mineral, or one of those amazing antioxidants. You can't even digest it. So just what is it, and why do cereal boxes brag about their fiber content?

Fiber is an indigestible carbohydrate found in plant-based foods like whole grains, legumes, vegetables, and fruits. In plants, these fibers keep cell walls strong and protect cellular contents. Dietary fiber helps to curb overeating, enables our digestive system to work smoothly, modulates the uptake of vitamins, minerals, and sugars from the stomach into the bloodstream and, in a little-appreciated function, promotes the health of our lower intestines. Studies over the past four decades show that diets high in fiber reduce rates of cardiovascular disease and diabetes, and help prevent constipation and a painful intestinal condition called diverticulitis. Numerous studies show fiber also battles obesity by promoting a feeling of satiety rivaling that of rich, high-fat meals. It may also play a role in preventing cancer.

People have long known that fiber is beneficial—remember the advice to get your roughage? That advice is now official, with leading health organizations recommending daily fiber consumption of 20 to 35 grams for adults. Most Americans, however, fall far short of this simple goal, eating about half that amount. And in doing so, they're falling short of reaching optimal health.

What Scientists Know

Fiber promotes good health by, in essence, slowing things down and then speeding them up. Foods high in fiber take longer to chew, and remain in your stomach longer. In your small intestine, fibers bind with cholesterol, lowering overall blood levels while improving your ratio of "good" to "bad" cholesterol. They also extend the absorption time of sugars in food, preventing the blood sugar spikes that can lead to diabetes. Once in the colon, fiber performs a seemingly odd function. It provides a short-term home and nourishment for the beneficial microflora living there, which actually keep your colon walls nourished and protected. From this point on, fiber accelerates the passage of solid waste from the body.

There are essentially two kinds of dietary fibers: soluble fibers that partially dissolve in water and insoluble fibers that don't. Each, in their own way, promotes gastrointestinal health.

Meals high in fiber provide strong protection against cardiovascular disease, according to years of research. Conclusive evidence shows that the soluble fibers in such foods as whole oats lower LDL cholesterol levels. And a 2004 federal study reported that dietary fibers result in lower levels of C-reactive protein, a blood marker linked to increased heart disease risk. In one study involving 40,000 men, researchers reported that those who ate the most dietary fiber decreased their odds of developing heart disease by a remarkable 40 percent. Other research finds connections between modest blood pressure declines and high fiber intake.

The influence of fiber in cancer prevention is less clear. In 2000, the medical establishment did an about-face regarding the protective effect of fiber against colon cancer after studies found a weak connection between high dietary fiber and a reduction in colon cancer rates. That reversed a decades-old conclusion that fiber served as a kind of colonic sweep, clearing out cancerous agents. But not everyone is convinced the link is tenuous. Not only is that counterintuitive, but a review by the World Cancer Research Fund of more than 4500 studies found that high consumption of dietary fiber—primarily from vegetables and cereals—played an important role in colon cancer prevention.

"The data on that is mixed but the overall good health of the intestinal tract would be protective against those types of diseases," says Joanne Slavin,

PhD, RD, a food science and nutrition professor at the University of Minnesota.

One of the less appreciated benefits of fiber centers on its highly effective role in controlling appetite and weight. "We know that people who eat more fiber weigh less, there's just very clear data," Slavin says. Not only do fiber-rich foods tend to take longer to eat, but they also absorb water during their journey through the gastrointestinal tract, promoting a feeling of fullness.

Making It Real

Multigrain cereals, wheat bran, brown rice, oatmeal, and popcorn are excellent sources of fiber, as are oranges, pears, apples, prunes, berries, broccoli, and beans.

To reach the recommended levels of 20 to 35 grams per day of fiber, start the day with a bowl of bran-based cereal (14 grams for Fiber One), and have an orange on the side (3 grams). For lunch, enjoy a sandwich with two slices of whole wheat bread (5 grams), with a cup of strawberries for a mid-afternoon snack (3 grams). At dinner, include a bowl of whole wheat pasta (9 grams), and you're at 34 grams.

Slavin says people often take a fiber supplement like Metamucil rather than change their diet, but she says it's not the same as whole foods. Nutritionists, Slavin includes, repeatedly state that bona fide foods—not supplements—are the best way to get fiber, as foods also contain a plethora of vitamins, minerals and phyto-chemicals that work synergistically. "Real foods have real advantages," Slavin says.

Increase your fiber intake slowly to give your gut a chance to adjust. Be sure to drink plenty of water as you add fiber to your diet. This takes advantage of fiber's ability to absorb water and promotes a feeling of fullness.

To Learn More

Visit the Harvard University's School of Public Health website at www.hsph.harvard.edu/nutritionsource and select the "Fiber" icon.

CHAPTER 30

Choose your Fish Carefully

In 1970, Danish researchers noticed a startling paradox in a settlement of Eskimos in Greenland. These people usually ate a pound a day of whale and seal meat, with fish and game served on the side. Hardly your ordinary balanced diet.

What amazed the researchers was the Inuits' virtual absence of heart disease in the face of this high-fat, high-cholesterol bill of fare. During a four-year period, only two people died of heart attacks among the 1,300 residents. Inflammatory diseases like arthritis were also almost nonexistent.

These findings challenged the medical dogma that excess dietary fat and cholesterol clog arteries and lead to premature death from heart disease. Clearly, something was protecting these people from the dangers of saturated fats and cholesterol. That mysterious agent turned out to be omega-3 fatty acids, which are found in abundance in marine life.

Since then, thousands of studies have reported on the benefits of regular fish consumption, including protection against heart disease, stroke, Alzheimer's disease, arthritis and numerous cancers.

But this good news about fish consumption and its role in promoting health has taken a disturbing twist, as toxicologists report that a significant portion of the world's seafood is contaminated with pollutants like mercury and PCBs. Suddenly, seafood meals come served with a dilemma: Eat too much, and you could literally poison yourself. But don't eat any, and you're at increased risk for a number of chronic diseases.

Jane Hightower, MD, a San Francisco internist who made international news when she reported that many of her patients suffered from mercury poisoning from fish consumption, advocates teaching consumers to make smart choices about which fish to eat, and how often. That's an obligation, she adds, that public health organizations have fallen short in fulfilling.

"The Food and Drug Administration certainly hasn't done much to educate the consumer," she says. "If you can't eat any food substance every day, you should be warned."

What Scientists Know

Investigations into seafood's health effect follow two paths: one studies the health benefits of a diet high in fish, while the other examines its dangers.

The strongest data on its benefits supports the Danish researchers' initial observation: Fish consumption protects the heart. A 2004 study reported that, compared with those who rarely or never ate fish, deaths from coronary heart disease declined 11 percent in those eating fish 1 to 3 times a month, while dropping 38 percent in people eating fish at least 5 times a week. Another 2004 study found that consuming fish just 1 to 3 times a month lowered rates of stroke. It's linked to lowered blood pressure and triglyceride levels, both risk factors for heart disease. Omega-3 fatty acids also protect cardiovascular health by preventing blood platelets from sticking together and forming clots, or adhering to artery walls and triggering plaque buildup.

These remarkable fish oils also reduce rates of autoimmune disorders like rheumatoid arthritis. Omega-3 fatty acids help prevent diabetes and ameliorate depression. The fish oils may also protect against cancers of the mouth, esophagus, stomach, colon, rectum, pancreas and prostate. The influence of omega-3 fatty acids in breast cancer prevention is inconclusive, although populations regularly eating fish, like the Japanese and the Inuit, have lower rates.

But, in one of the stranger sagas in medical research, scientists are learning that the pollutants accumulated in fish can offset its health benefits. A 2002 study reported that mercury in fish cancelled out its heart-protective effects. Research on primates linked mercury consumption with miscarriages and lowered reproductive capacity in both sexes. It's also a potent neurotoxin, causing cognitive impairment.

Mercury can trigger an autoimmune response, Hightower says, which may explain some chronic maladies in patients that defy diagnoses, like fatigue, memory lapses, hair loss, headaches, and muscle and joint pains. In the patients she studied, whom she selected because of their affinity for seafood or because they had symptoms of mercury poisoning, she found that 90 percent had mercury levels exceeding federal safe levels—some more than seventeen-fold. After they stopped eating fish, their symptoms faded.

PCBs may amplify the effects of mercury. Studies have also found direct connections between PCB exposure and the development of cancer, immune system and neurological impairment, and reproductive harm.

Making It Real

Omega-3 fatty acids are too important to forego eating fish due to fears of contaminants. Some researchers believe that omega-3 fatty acids may actually be essential to preventing many chronic diseases. "It's a very sad scenario," Hightower comments, that a food of such value is so tainted by pollution. But she adds that there are ways to enjoy fish without undue exposure to mercury or PCBs.

First, avoid or limit consumption of fish high on the food chain—the predatory fish. Mercury ascends the food chain from small to large fish, becoming more concentrated with each step. Avoid swordfish, mackerel and shark altogether. Albacore tuna shouldn't be eaten more than once a week. Chunk light tuna can be eaten twice weekly, as it comes from younger tuna with relatively low mercury exposure.

Non-predatory coldwater fish like salmon, trout, herring and sardines contain high levels of omega-3 fatty acids, and are low in mercury. Shrimp, crab, anchovies, catfish, herring, mackerel, oysters, clams, and lobster are also relatively low in mercury. (All fish contain at least trace amounts of this heavy metal.) Since PCBs accumulate in fatty tissue, cut away skin and fat before cooking fish. Mercury, unfortunately, is tightly bound in muscle cells, and can't be cooked out.

To Learn More

The Physicians for Social Responsibility has a "Healthy Fish, Healthy Families" guide on its website at www.mercuryaction.org/fish. You can also order the guide by calling (202) 667-4260.

CHAPTER 31

Avoid Alzheimer's

When most people ponder their health and fitness, they're thinking about their shoulders on down. Experts in dementia would like you to think otherwise. "There was an assumption that as you got older, you get senile and there's nothing you can do about it. That it's a normal part of aging," says Gary Small, MD, the director of the Center on Aging at the University of California, Los Angeles and author of *The Memory Prescription*.

"Well, we've learned it's not necessarily normal," he continues, "and there are things you can do about it, not just in terms of medicines but in terms of lifestyle."

Don't feel chagrined if you haven't considered how to feed and care for the brain. Public education campaigns on maintaining brain health are almost nonexistent, in contrast to other chronic diseases. Yet almost five million Americans have Alzheimer's disease, twice the number of people with cardiovascular disease.

The greatest risk factor for Alzheimer's disease is advanced age. But a recent crop of studies shows that the onset of dementia is also clearly linked to those tragically familiar health maladies—diabetes, obesity, high blood pressure, and cardiovascular disease.

This new knowledge is empowering people to care for their brains as well as their brawn. "Baby boomers tend to be proactive," notes Small. "They want to take charge of their future brain fitness and live a healthy brain lifestyle."

What Scientists Know

In 1906, Alois Alzheimer, a German psychiatrist, discovered the source of a disease that would one day bear his name: a damaging accumulation of protein fragments called amyloid plaques in the brain, as well as abnormally tangled nerve fibers. Alzheimer's disease is characterized by an annihilation of memory, and is the most prevalent form of dementia.

What remains unanswered is just what triggers the brain to go so wrong. But scientists are certain that the scourges of modern society play a significant role in the onset of Alzheimer's disease.

Stroke victims have an increased probability of developing Alzheimer's disease by more than 20 percent, according to one study. Heart disease also raises the risk, as does high blood pressure. Research shows that obesity can double or even triple the odds of developing

Alzheimer's. Another study found that those with diabetes faced a two-thirds increased risk of developing the disease, perhaps because of impaired uptake of insulin by brain cells. Chronic stress doubled the odds of developing Alzheimer's disease in a study of 800 men.

As if all that's not sobering enough, if you have two or more of these chronic conditions, the odds against you multiply. But scientists now have hard data showing that interventions against conditions like heart disease, stroke, and obesity also lower rates of Alzheimer's and other forms of dementia. Studies report that use of cholesterol-lowering statins reduces the likelihood of developing Alzheimer's. Intake of folic acid and vitamins B6 and B12, which lower homocysteine levels and hence reduce cardiovascular disease risk, appears to also protect against brain cell loss. In an encouraging advance, regular aspirin use is also linked to lower Alzheimer's rates in preliminary studies. In addition, people supplementing with 500 mg of vitamin C and 400 IUs of vitamin E cut their risk of developing the dementia by one-third, according to another study.

One of the least expensive and most enjoyable ways to keep Alzheimer's at bay by regularly exercising. One large study found that just walking 90 minutes a week reduced cognitive decline by 20 percent.

It's no exaggeration to call omega-3 fatty acids "brain food." Multiple studies show these fatty acids, found in salmon and other coldwater fish, boost long-term brain health. Eating fish once a week reduced the onset of

Alzheimer's disease by a whopping 60 percent, according to one study.

Regular tea drinking and moderate wine consumption also appear to lower the risk of Alzheimer's onset. A diet high in vegetables and low in meats is also protective, according to studies. Blueberries also provide powerful protection against Alzheimer's, according to numerous studies.

An intriguing 2005 study from UCLA also strongly suggests that curcumin, the pigment that gives curry its yellow color, helps prevent the buildup of amyloid plaque and may even destroy it, perhaps through curcumin's potent anti-inflammatory and antioxidant properties. Previous research on animals and populations in India support the hypothesis that curry is linked to lower rates of Alzheimer's disease.

An active social life plays a important role in preventing Alzheimer's, according to a review of major studies, as does engaging in mentally stimulating activities like playing chess and card games, or holding down a challenging job.

Making It Real

Given the ties between brain health and well-known chronic diseases, the advice for preventing personality-destroying dementias is familiar: maintain a normal weight, remain physically and socially active, eat sensibly, and even savor a glass of wine occasionally, if you're so inclined. Says Small on preventing dementia: "Living a healthy lifestyle and trying to address each of those four major areas—diet, mental activity, physical activity, and stress—will probably have a big impact."

The Alzheimer's Association's dementia-prevention advice includes: reduce your intake of saturated fats and cholesterol; fit physical activity into your daily schedule; consume dark leafy vegetables like spinach or romaine lettuce, and cruciferous vegetables like broccoli and Swiss chard frequently; choose fruits with high antioxidant levels like prunes, raisins, and blueberries; don't let a week go by without eating one or more servings of fish containing beneficial omega-3 fatty acids, such as halibut, salmon, or trout. While large-scale human tests of the brain-saving effect of curcumin haven't begun, curry is harmless. So feel free to enhance your anti-dementia arsenal by adding the spice to your diet. Also, take a multivitamin, in part to assure you're getting enough folic acid, which keeps homocysteine levels in check, and supplement with vitamins C and E. Maintain an active social life that includes mentally stimulating activities, and, if you're so disposed, keep working late into life.

To Learn More

Visit the Alzheimer's Association's website at www.alz.org or call its 24-hour National Call Center for information about Alzheimer's disease and related dementias at (800) 272-3900. Also visit the National Institute of Aging's website at www.alzheimers.org.

CHAPTER 32

Toast to Your Health

Hippocrates, the 4th century BC Greek physician, was among the first healers to prescribe wine for promoting health. Thomas Jefferson in 1818 railed against a heavy tax on wine, describing it as "a tax on the health of our citizens."

Now, hundreds of studies generated over the last 40 years provide solid evidence for one of humanity's most enduring hunches. The most famous is "The French Paradox," published in 1992 in the prestigious journal *Lancet*. The news show *60 Minutes* catapulted the scholarly study to fame after describing the researchers' conclusions: The French, despite enjoying a diet laden with butter, cheese, foie gras and other saturated animal fats, have low rates of cardiovascular disease, perhaps attributable to their daily habit of wine drinking.

That habit never took hold in America because of a more ambivalent attitude toward drinking. One U.S. researcher wrote in a memoir that federal health officials

in 1972 forbade publication of his work on wine's beneficial influence on heart health, citing the "socially unde-
sirable" nature of his conclusions.

Concerns about misuse of alcohol aren't misplaced,
health experts emphasize. Abusers of alcohol often die
prematurely, and have heaped countless heartaches on
their families as well as victims of alcohol-fueled accidents and violence.

But Arthur Klatsky, MD, a cardiologist with Kaiser
Permanente in Oakland, California, and a pioneering
researcher on alcohol's medical effects, says most people
who drink do so moderately. And with almost one million people dying annually in the United States from cardiovascular disease, many people may be unaware of one
nature's best medicines for prolonging their life.

Even Shakespeare wrote in defense of wine, when in
Othello he penned, "Come, come, good wine is a good
familiar creature if it be well used; exclaim no more
against it."

What Scientists Know

Light alcohol use helps prevent cardiovascular disease by
increasing levels of HDL cholesterol. These "good" cholesterols act as shuttles as they carry dangerous LDL cholesterols in blood and plaque back to the liver for
reprocessing. Alcohol also appears to makes blood
platelets less "sticky," and thus less prone to clotting or to

accumulating on artery walls. It may stimulate the production of an enzyme that breaks blood clots apart.

This blood-thinning and plaque-prevention activity of alcohol has its most dramatic effect in lowering rates of coronary artery disease. This disease is caused by plaque clogging the arteries that feed the heart with its own blood supply. When too much plaque accumulates, less blood reaches the heart, causing angina, or chest pain, as the heart muscle struggles with reduced oxygen and nutrients. Plaque fragments can also block coronary arteries, triggering a heart attack. Or plaque can block the blood vessels leading to the brain, causing an ischemic stroke. Numerous studies have confirmed alcohol's protective effect against plaque development and clot formation. In a 2003 study, Klatsky and colleagues report that an analysis involving almost 129,000 people found that those consuming one or two drinks daily had a 32 percent lower risk of dying of coronary heart disease than abstainers. And a Danish study with more than 13,000 participants finds that those drinking wine daily, weekly, or even monthly had a significantly lower risk of ischemic stroke, compared to nondrinkers. Alcohol's role in stroke prevention may also explain the results of a headline-grabbing 2002 study which reported that moderate drinkers had a 42 percent reduction for all types of dementia, including Alzheimer's disease, compared with abstainers. "You might expect that alcohol would be protective against dementia caused by multiple small strokes, because most of them are ischemic strokes," explains Klatsky. A 2005 study also reports that, among elderly women, nondrinkers had greater cognitive decline than moderate drinkers.

Light alcohol consumption may lower rates of LDL oxidation, a process that also causes plaque buildup. Klatsky says it might actually be the action of antioxidants and other phytochemicals abundant in wines, dark beers, and hard ciders that prevent LDL oxidation—compounds that can also be found in non-alcoholic foods like grape juice or fruits. Moderate drinking also appears to lessen insulin resistance, a risk factor for diabetes, which in turn often increases plaque buildup. "Diabetes is strongly associated with atherosclerosis, all over the body," Klatsky says.

Wine, beer, and hard liquor all seem to protect against cardiovascular disease, although studies vary as to the effectiveness of each. But factors like phytochemicals in the beverage or lifestyle differences between people favoring one drink over another may affect study outcomes.

Making It Real

If you already drink in moderation, you can do so knowing you're giving your health a lift. Moderate is defined as one drink a day for women, or up to two a day for men. Amounts beyond that begin to reverse the health benefits, such as increasing rates of several types of cancer, diabetes, high blood pressure, dementia and hemorrhagic stroke—the kind caused by bleeding in the brain. "Because a little bit may be good for you doesn't mean more is better," Klatsky emphasizes. It's also best to drink with meals, he says, as it evens out blood alcohol levels. There's also preliminary evidence that drinking without food may slightly elevate blood pressure.

And all health experts emphasize responsible drinking, which includes not driving after drinking, or binge drinking.

But you should steer clear of alcohol if you or a close family member has a history of problems with alcohol use. You can pursue comparable health benefits through other avenues, like exercising and eating an abundance of fruits, vegetables, and whole grains. However, if you stopped light drinking because you thought it might harm your health, you may want to rethink that position. As Klatsky says, given all the known health benefits of light drinking, "That self-imposed prohibition should be repealed."

To Learn More

Visit the website of Alcohol in Moderation, or AIM, a group promoting responsible consumption of alcohol, at www.aim-digest.com.

CHAPTER 33

Watch Your Back

While back problems won't kill you, the pain may make you wish you were dead. Few maladies are more disruptive to the quality of a person's life than back pain. Only colds and the flu account for more doctor visits and time off from work than back problems. Eight out of ten people will experience severe back pain at some point in their lives.

As with maintaining strong legs, one of the most important steps you can take to ensure mobility and independence late into life is to strengthen and protect your back now.

Back pain, among the most excruciating that a person can experience, can circumscribe your life and lead to surgery, immobility, permanent disability, and depression. These complications can ultimately shorten your life span, not to mention degrade the quality of your life.

Fortunately, there's much you can do to protect your back. If professional football has demonstrated anything, it's that with proper muscle development, the human back can endure almost any insult. No activity, by its very nature, routinely imparts greater physical stress on the back. One need only view the bone-crunching hits and the bodily contortions that follow when 250-pound men collide at full speed. Yet with rare exceptions, they get up, trot back to the huddle, and repeat the process the next play. The ferocity of the impact would immobilize the average person. Yet professional football players rarely miss time from work because of back pain, due to a strong armor of muscles protecting them from injury. That's a strategy we can all adopt.

What Scientists Know

The spine is made up of 33 interlocking bones called vertebras, each stacked upon the next at a slight angle to form the spine's S-shaped curve. Each vertebra is separated from the next by a flexible pad of tissue that cushions the vertebras and prevents them from grinding against each other. These bones are then held in place by an intricate system of muscles and ligaments.

But ultimately it's the muscles of the back and stomach that protect the integrity of the spine. This is the musculature professional athletes have developed that enables them to endure the abuse on the field and keep performing for years.

Strong muscles in the stomach and the back are the single best way to avoid back problems. Strong muscles support the spine, distribute the weight of the body evenly, and absorb routine stresses from movement. In contrast, weak muscles don't support weight of the body, instead transferring the load to the spinal column. Over time, this can lead to vertebral disc degeneration and chronic pain. Weak muscles are also more susceptible to sprains and spasms, both among the leading causes of lower back pain.

According to Mark Brown, MD, with the University of Miami Medical School, the main cause of back pain is being out of shape. In a study of firefighters, he notes that those who exercise regularly had fewer and less severe attacks of back pain, compared with non-exercisers.

Although exercises which strengthen stomach or back muscles directly benefit back health, researchers now know that even aerobic exercise helps by improving blood circulation to the back muscles and discs. Strong legs and flexible hamstrings also support back health, as they bear more of the burden of heavy lifting and moving about.

Obesity can certainly lead to back problems. The additional weight taxes muscles, tendons, and ligaments. The additional weight also discourages the practice of performing back-preserving exercises. Numerous studies have shown that losing weight is a key avenue to better back health.

Maintaining good posture, one that avoids slouching, leaning or otherwise losing the S-shaped curve in the back, helps prevent back problems. Arthur White, MD, former president of the Spine Society and the author of *The Posture Prescription*, notes that just by standing and sitting with good posture, we maintain the optimum alignment of the bones and the discs in the back. Simple exercises like leaning against a wall and holding your shoulders back can help maintain healthy spine alignment.

Chronic back pain disrupts one's life in myriad ways. Sleep becomes difficult, moving about challenging, and performing work difficult or impossible. Not surprisingly, chronic back pain is also a significant source of major depression, according to studies.

While many of the causes of back pain are obvious, such as overexertion and incorrect lifting, others aren't. Research shows that people who smoke have more back pain, as it appears that compounds in tobacco smoke interfere with blood oxygen levels and in the delivery of nutrients to back muscles and discs. Smoking has also been shown to increase sensitivity to pain, probably because of nicotine's effect on the brain.

Making It Real

By far the best way to enjoy a lifetime free of debilitating back pain is to prevent it. Muscle strength, weight control and proper use of the back in lifting and moving are all essential to maintaining back health. Every exercise routine should include strength training for the abdominal muscles, such as sit-ups and crunches.

Go for overall strength in your exercise routine, but be sure to include exercises for your lower back, such as back extensions, yoga, and stretches.

To avoid one of the leading triggers for back pain, learn how to properly lift heavy objects by making certain your spine remain perpendicular to the floor and your legs bear most of the load. And while weight belts provide a sense of security, studies are decidedly mixed on their effectiveness.

A personal trainer or a book on back health will provide ample exercises to develop back strength. Remember to drink plenty of water to help to maintain disc hydration.

To Learn More

For comprehensive information on back health, visit www.spine-health.com. The doctor-run, noncommercial website features a series of easy-to-read articles on prevention and treatment of back pain.

CHAPTER 34

Eat Less Meat

The largest and most powerful primate on the planet, and one of our nearest evolutionary cousins, is vegetarian. The gorilla, which can grow to more than 400 pounds, supports itself by eating roots, leaves, shoots, and fruits. Perhaps there's a lesson here.

Other chapters have stressed the importance of eating multiple servings of whole grains, copious quantities of fruits, and a bounty of vegetables. As a corollary, it's also important to consider eating less meat to achieve optimal health.

We're a meat-centered culture, despite the fact that meat is often loaded with saturated fat and cholesterol, generally calorie-dense, and taxing on the body to digest. Multiple studies have demonstrated that vegetarians live longer and have overall better health than those who rely upon meat as a mainstay in their diet. Contrary to the popular myth, a diet based upon a variety of plant sources easily provides sufficient levels of protein to maintain muscle and tissue health.

Diets high in meat are not as nutritionally neutral as once thought. Studies now link them to heart disease, stroke, osteoporosis and some forms of cancer. They're also one of the reasons our population is among the most obese in the world.

Our love affair with meat is no doubt a product of relatively cheap prices, convenience, taste preferences, and ironically concerns about adequate nutrition. It's also the result of the ever-present and powerful promotion by the companies who market our meat and poultry products. Their influence is not only reflected in the media, but surfaces in schools and the government agencies charged with protecting our food and shaping our diets. Meat has become as American as apple pie.

It's time to separate the meat from the chaff.

What Scientists Know

Americans consume nearly twice the level of protein they actually need for health, and the vast majority of the excess comes from animal sources, often red meat.

According to Walter Willett, MD, with the Harvard School of Public Health, the average woman needs no more than 50 grams of protein per day, and the average man, 65 grams. But can people take in adequate levels of protein on a plant-based diet?

The American Dietetic Association and the Dieticians of Canada set out to answer this and other questions about vegetarian diets. Their detailed 2003 report concludes that "plant protein can meet the requirement for adequate protein when a variety of plants are consumed." Even athletes can meet their demands for protein on plant-based diets, they notes. Many vegetables, such as beans, nuts, and even spinach are high in protein. In fact, calorie for calorie, spinach provides as much protein as prime rib.

High-protein, meat-centered diets can pose a serious health hazard in the long term. Two recent studies demonstrated that when the body metabolizes high levels of animal protein, it draws upon stores of calcium in the body to neutralize the proteins' acidity. Much of this calcium comes directly from the bone, and the mineral is later excreted. Many researchers now conclude that this phenomenon explains why populations in the United States and Scandinavia, with their high consumption of animal protein and dairy products, still have high rates of osteoporosis. Populations in Japan and China, where meat is served as a side dish, have very low rates of this bone-wasting disease.

Diets high in meat, particularly red meat, are directly implicated in increased incidence of heart disease and stroke, due in large part to the cholesterol and saturated fat inherent in such bills of fare. Overly generous servings of meat also displace health-promoting foods like vegetables and whole grains on the plate. Certain cancers, such as prostate cancer, develop more frequently among populations relying upon red meat. People who build their diets around meat also tend to be significantly heavier that those eating little or no meat. And a landmark study of a religious denomination with a large number of vegetarians found that those who ate meat for many years were more than three times as likely to develop signs of dementia, compared with their non-meat-eating counterparts.

Major health research organizations, including the American Cancer Society, the American Institute for Cancer Research, and Harvard School of Public Health, all recommend a rethinking of our reliance upon meat as a dietary staple. Each recommends plant-based diets with limited consumption of meat protein. The Harvard School of Public Health has even devised its own alternative food pyramid, which places red meat at the pinnacle of the pyramid, emphasizing limited consumption.

Making It Real

The point of this research is to illustrate that you can easily get by with less meat, and to underscore the advantages of a diet predominated by fruits, vegetables, nuts, and grains. The era of ham and eggs for breakfast, a burger for lunch, and a steak for dinner appears to be fading in the face of urgings by health experts to ease up on our meat habit.

The first step is to rethink the size of meat portions and the frequency with which you eat meat. Wean yourself from the 10-ounce slab of meat, and experiment with

3-ounce portions. Try eating meat at most once a day, or even cutting back to a few times a week. Consider following a vegetarian diet for a day or two, or even a week, and see how you feel. (You may even lose weight.) Or combine small morsels of meat, chicken, or fish in vegetables dishes, as is typical of many Asian and Mediterranean cuisines. There are countless books and websites to guide you to interesting and delicious recipes.

To Learn More

Visit the Harvard School of Public Health's "Food Pyramids: What Should You Really Eat?" website at www.hsph. harvard.edu/nutritionsource/pyramids.html.

CHAPTER 35

Win the Weight War

The Old Amish Order in southern Ontario provides a revealing glimpse back at our far more physically active—and slender—past. The followers of this religious order, who eschew modern technologies like cars and electrical appliances, are six times as active as most Americans, and obesity is rare among them. Yet the Amish enjoy three meals a day, with foods like eggs, meat, potatoes, gravy, vegetables, breads, pies, and cakes. It's their level of physical activity, researchers studying the group concluded, that keeps the Amish fit.

Today, half of Americans don't achieve even minimum recommended levels of physical activity, and 16 percent are inactive, according to federal statistics. It's no surprise, then, that almost two-thirds of Americans are overweight. But these staggering statistics don't simply reflect a lack of discipline on the part of Americans; they also reveal the profound influence of labor-saving technologies and aggressive food marketing.

Suburban sprawl promotes weight gain, as people become more reliant on their cars. City dwellers, studies show, walk more and are on average thinner than those in suburbs. Remote controls, the Internet, and computer games keep children and adults seat-bound for hours. Even small acts of exertion, like opening a garage door or raking leaves, are no longer necessary, thanks to the advent of machines that do the job. And to a degree unparalleled in history, high-fat, low-fiber foods—served in mega-portions—abound in restaurants and supermarkets.

It's a daunting goal to remain slender in modern times, one that requires adopting a smart strategy for countering the many factors that promote growing girth.

What Scientists Know

Hypertension, high cholesterol, diabetes, asthma, arthritis, and certain cancers are triggered or worsened by excess weight, as are psychological problems like depression and low self-esteem. Studies show even modest weight loss improves this bleak picture, by ameliorating these conditions and increasing life span.

While regular physical activity is essential for maintaining permanent weight loss, it's virtually impossible to shed pounds without first changing your food choices. That's why weight loss is so difficult, as most diets require that people cut out favorite foods, restrict portions to unsatisfying small sizes, or lose weight on an unsustainable bill of fare.

But there is an effective strategy to permanently lose weight that doesn't require calorie counting, and that allows you to eat the foods you enjoy while enhancing your health with nutritious fare. It's built on the principle that people need to feel satiated after meals for successful weight loss. You achieve that by filling up on water-rich foods like vegetables, soups and fruits while enjoying smaller portions of the richer foods you love. It's a diet described in *The Volumetrics Eating Plan*, written by Barbara Rolls, PhD, an authority on successful weight loss and a professor of nutritional science at Pennsylvania State University.

Rolls describes these water-rich foods as "low in energy density;" in other words, low in calories for the volume of the serving. In contrast, foods with low water content are high in energy density. For example, a quarter cup of raisins—an energy-dense food—contains 100 calories and is equivalent to almost two cups of grapes. Yet after consuming the grapes, you'll probably feel more satisfied than you would by eating the raisins. In one study Rolls conducted, participants eating chicken soup were more quickly satiated and ate less during the meal than those who consumed the identical ingredients and the same amount of food in a thicker chicken casserole. One study she worked on found that people who chose low density foods actually ate more and lost more weight than those eating higher density foods. "If you're choosing low energy density foods, you're going to get a lot more food. And our data shows you're likely to be a lot more satisfied," Rolls says.

Making It Real

The beauty of emphasizing low-density, water-rich foods like vegetables and fruits in your meals is that you don't have to cut out any of your cherished foods. You just need to serve smaller portions of them. For example, in her earlier book, *The Volumetrics Weight-Control Plan*, Rolls states that when she's at a buffet, she piles her plate with greens and fruits, and spoons a modest amount of dressing on the side. Rolls then takes small scoops of a variety of foods, so she can enjoy richer entrees and side dishes, as well as dessert. But by filling up on the low-density, fiber-rich foods, she becomes more satiated and less inclined to overeat.

Being tempted with a wide variety of foods is another trigger for overeating, she says. That's why diets that rely on a narrow range of choices, like the cabbage soup diet, work; you get tired of the same foods and lose your appetite. But even satiated diners' appetites perk up when an enticing new dish arrives. To cope with this tendency to overeat when faced with an array of choices, Rolls suggests providing yourself with an assortment of flavorful low-density foods, like seasoned vegetables, mixed fruit salad, or broth-based soups.

Consuming soup at the start of a meal is an excellent way to prevent overeating. In a study Rolls presented at a 2004 scientific meeting, she reported that people eating soup lost more weight than those eating the equivalent number of calories as snack foods, and kept it off. In

Volumetrics, Rolls explains that with soup, two cups can be equivalent in calories to a serving of crackers and cheese, yet the soup is much more filling. In addition, the aroma and the sensation of eating this flavorful food add to the satisfaction it provides.

To Learn More

For information on nutrition and physical activity, visit the National Center for Chronic Disease Prevention and Health Promotion's website at www.cdc.gov/nccdphp/dnpa/nutrition.htm.

CHAPTER 36

Downsize Your Plate

It's not just a lack of exercise or ineffective weight loss programs that are keeping Americans frustratingly out-of-shape. It's also our distorted perception of what constitutes normal food servings.

Over the past 20 years, bagels doubled in size to 6-inch handfuls, fast-food cheeseburgers swelled by 257 calories, and a bottle of soda increased from 6.5 ounces to 20 ounces. Restaurants are responding to American's enthusiasm for mega-sized portions by serving up meals that could feed two or even three diners. A slab of ribs at a Houlihan's restaurant contains more than twice the protein suggested by the federal government for a single serving, and 7 times the number of french fries. Bigger portions are now even dished out in American homes. A national survey of food consumption patterns between 1977 and 1996 found an upward trend in serving sizes for meals prepared at home, similar to that seen in restaurants and fast-food outlets.

So how are diners responding to the super-sizing of their meals? Apparently by keeping pace and cleaning their plates, no matter how absurdly large the servings. Studies show that when presented with outsized meals, people finish them, yet feel no more satisfaction than when they ate smaller amounts. Americans now consume on average 150 more calories per day than they did 20 years ago, which can translate into a 15-pound weight gain annually. "Most individuals eat all or most of what is served," says Barbara Rolls, PhD, an expert on food portions and satiety, and a professor of nutritional science at Pennsylvania State University. "The excess food in mega-portions isn't going home in doggy bags; it is, instead, fueling the obesity epidemic."

Portion control is the new focus of nutritionists and health officials alarmed at the consequences of growing girth. And the National Institutes of Health and major health organizations are pushing initiatives to help Americans recognize proper portion sizes.

What Scientists Know

Eating most or even all of a 12-inch sandwich wasn't significantly more satiating than eating an entire 8-inch sandwich, researchers at Pennsylvania State University found. Yet the women enrolled in their study on average ate 74 more calories when eating the larger sandwich, and men an additional 186 calories. In another experiment,

Penn State researchers reported that as portion sizes served over a two-day period increased, men and women participating in the study just ate more; they didn't compensate for the excess by cutting back the next meal. When portion sizes were doubled, the women ate 530 more calories per day and men ate 803 more. "Most people, even when we double portions, don't even notice it," says Rolls.

Yet decreasing the caloric density of foods didn't lead to a decreased sense of fullness or satiety, another study reported. Researchers found that men and women given large portions of cheesy pasta made less calorie-dense with added vegetables felt just as satiated as when they ate a same-sized portion of a richer version, loaded with more cheese but fewer vegetables. Rolls notes that the study supported the conclusion that chefs can prepare lower-calorie fare without creating customer dissatisfaction.

But not all hefty portions are implicated in weight gain. Some, in fact, do the opposite. "Low energy density foods," like soups, lettuce, and fruits, contain a high percentage of water. Thus, per unit volume, they contain fewer calories than foods like cheese, meats, and pastas. Research conducted by Rolls concluded that diners who consumed a large first course of low density foods, like a soup or a lightly dressed salad, ate up to 12 percent less during the meal than those who didn't start with such light fare. Piling your plate high with fresh salad greens or seasoned vegetables, or enjoying a savory bowl of soup, may be among the best weight loss strategies. "Any big volume of a low density food is going to give you a lot of sensory satisfaction," Rolls notes. It also facilitates weight loss by emphasizing "positive messages rather than negative, restrictive messages," she adds.

Making It Real

The best strategy to avoid overeating is to steer clear of large portions of calorie-dense foods. "You need to be aware that if you have a big portion of food in front of you, it's likely you're going to eat more," Rolls says. At restaurants, share an entrée or ask if half orders are available. You can also order an appetizer, which often provides a normal serving under USDA guidelines. And if you do order soup, avoid high-calorie, cream-based broths.

Become familiar with the federal guidelines for portion sizes, and use them to recalibrate your view of what constitutes a single serving. A half cup of rice or pasta is a serving, but many restaurant entrees contain at least four times that amount. One nutritionist suggests measuring out foods for a few days, following the measurements on food labels (which reflect federal guidelines) for a single serving. Then make a mental note of what a single serving looks like.

At home, be aware of the tendency to prepare extra food when you've got a large container of ingredients. Also, don't eat directly from a box; pull out an allocated

amount and exercise your willpower to not eat more.
(Willpower, like muscle, gets stronger the more you use
it.) And don't serve meals family style. Instead, serve
meals in the kitchen and don't return for seconds. Use
smaller plates as well. Studies show that the larger the
plate, the larger the portions served.

To Learn More

Click on "The New American" plate icon on the website of the
American Institute for Cancer Research at www.aicr.org. The
institute, which supports research on diet and its role in cancer prevention, offers simple strategies for filling your plate
with foods that promote health and keep the extra pounds
from piling on.

Also visit the National Institutes of Health's "Portion
Distortion" website at http://hin.nhlbi.nih.gov/portion.

CHAPTER 37

Rest Your Weary Soul

Thomas Edison's invention of the incandescent bulb in 1879 ushered in a glowing new age, but brought with it an unintended consequence: The modern era of chronic sleep deprivation. In our brightly illuminated and hyperactive world, the normal rhythm of sleep that evolved with the setting and rising of the sun rarely return except during wilderness excursions.

Sleep deprivation is endemic in our culture. In the 19th century, people slept 10 hours a night. Today, Americans average 6.9 hours of sleep on weeknights and 7.5 hours per night on weekends, according to a National Sleep Foundation poll. William C. Dement, MD, the founder of Stanford University's Sleep Research Center, the world's first sleep disorder research institute, regards America as a "sleep-sick society."

Most people try to cram too much activity into each day. But shaving off a couple of hours of sleep to fit in more work or fun is a poor trade-off in health, mood, and even longevity. Studies show that chronic sleep deprivation is linked with increased risk of hypertension, chronic stress, diabetes, and cardiovascular disease and may even promote obesity by altering hormone levels. It's linked to cognitive impairment such as a decline in reaction time, judgment, logical reasoning, verbal ability, short-term memory and decision-making ability. A good night's repose is a potent restorer of good cheer, while sleep deprivation leads to irritation, depression and other negative moods. Population studies also reveal that poor sleepers are much more likely to have health problems than sound sleepers. Dement is certain that tens of thousands of people in the United States die from undiagnosed sleep problems and their related complications.

Sleep deprivation is also the little-known culprit behind countless tragic accidents. The federal government estimates that driver fatigue leads to at least 100,000 crashes and more than 1,500 deaths yearly. Fatigue played a role in the Exxon Valdez oil spill, the Challenger space shuttle explosion, and the Chernobyl and Three Mile Island nuclear plant accidents, investigators concluded.

What Scientists Know

Sleep is a mysterious process that's still poorly understood. But what is known that while sleeping, rapid-eye movement and slow wave sleep both play complementary roles in memory consolidation, which is the process of imprinting memories in your brain. Research reveals impairment of short-term memory with sleep deficits. A sound snooze can also promote faster problem-solving skills. Research with students showed that those getting adequate rest were twice as likely to figure out the short-cut to a math problem, compared with the sleep-deprived.

Adults need between 7 and 9 hours of sleep per night; the amount varies by individual. You can determine your own optimal level simply by noting the length of sleep you need to feel alert and refreshed throughout the day, says Clete Kushida, MD, PhD, the director of Stanford's Center for Human Sleep Research. Any amount less than optimal begins to accumulate as a sleep debt. You can repay a short-term debt with extra sleep within a few days; however, after a significant sleep debt builds, your risk of developing conditions like high blood pressure and mood disorders increases. Another effect of sleep deprivation is immune system impairment, which can lead to increased risk of contracting infectious illnesses like the common cold.

Sleep apnea, which affects about 15 million Americans, is one of the more dangerous sleep disorders. Loud snoring is one manifestation of sleep apnea, a sound caused by a partial obstruction of airways. People with apnea often awaken due to inadequate oxygen intake, and their heart begins racing to increase their breathing rate, a reaction that raises blood pressure. These repetitive spikes in blood pressure can damage organs and blood vessels and can even induce small strokes.

About half of Americans cope with insomnia two or more times a week, according to the National Sleep Foundation. And roughly half of those cases are caused by worry and stress. The rest is chronic insomnia, which may be caused by sleep disorders such as apnea, restless legs syndrome, or gastroesophageal reflux. The latter two are also serious conditions, and require medical attention.

Making It Real

Strong light, like sunlight, is a powerful regulator of our biological clock, and by regulating your exposure, you can promote sounder sleep. Stanford's Kushida advises dimming lights two to three hours before going to bed. He also says 30 minutes of sun exposure in the morning helps synchronize your internal clock closer to nature's schedule. Housebound people, in fact, may develop sleep problems due to insufficient daytime light exposure.

Sleep experts strongly advise maintaining a regular sleep schedule, and following it even on the weekends. They also advise against naps, unless you feel tired and are about to undertake a hazardous endeavor or drive a vehicle. If you're getting adequate rest, you should remain alert throughout the entire day. Regular exercise, which reduces stress and anxiety, contributes to sound repose when completed at least three hours before bedtime. Of course, steer clear of beverages containing caffeine later in the day, as it can take six hours or longer to clear the stimulant from your brain. Don't engage in stimulating or vexing activities before bed, like watching an action film or the evening news, checking emails, or paying bills.

Kushida says the current generation of prescription sleep drugs is effective, and that there's "overconcern" that people will become addicted to them. Over-the-counter sleep aids rely on antihistamines, drugs that block activity of nerve cells, inducing sleep. But they can be less effective over time, and take longer to wear off. Studies show that supplements containing melatonin, a hormone that induces sleep, can help promote sound sleep.

If you snore, or feel persistent, strange sensations in your legs at night, you should see a sleep specialist. Do the same if chronic heartburn keeps you awake; it's a sign of gastroesophageal reflux, a dangerous condition that increases your risk of esophageal cancer.

To Learn More

Visit the National Sleep Foundation's website at www.sleepfoundation.org for extensive information on insomnia and other sleep disorders, as well as suggestions for enjoying a good night's rest.

CHAPTER 38

Keep the Faith

Recent findings that routine churchgoers live longer, healthier lives even has pragmatic scientists intrigued. "I'm not a very religious person, so I think I'd be the last to proclaim people go to church as a way to improve their health," says Robert Hummer, PhD, the director of the Population Center at the University of Texas at Austin. "But as a scientist, you look at this data and go 'wow, maybe there's something going on here.'"

Hummer, a prominent researcher on religion and its influence on health, has found that people who regularly attend church not only outlive those who don't, but have lower rates of chronic diseases. That's after accounting for other influences such as education and income, marital status, social networks outside of the congregation, health status, and avoiding behaviors considered sinful, like smoking or abusing alcohol. "It's showing up consistently. But what I think the field is really struggling with is why," Hummer says.

Scientists believe it reflects a confluence of factors, such as the sense of acceptance shared by fellow congregation members, urgings to follow healthful practices, and encouragement to get married and stay that way. Congregation members also provide practical support to one another, such as helping with chores, providing transportation, and assisting with finances. Religious followers also find comfort in relinquishing problems through prayer, Hummer says. This unburdening provides relief from worry and stress that few in the secular world know.

What Scientists Know

Most of the research on religion and health shows that regular attendance of religious services lengthens lives. In one study involving 21,000 adults, Hummer and colleagues found that attending religious services more than once a week was linked to a seven-year increase in life span. Those who never attended a service were also four times more likely to die of a respiratory or infectious disease. Another researcher analyzed 28 years of data of more than 2,600 people in Alameda County in Northern California, and reported that those who attended a church or temple at least weekly were more likely to have good mental health, a wider social circle and a stable marriage. Other research has also linked regular religious attendance with good mental health, in particular significantly lowered rates of depression and anxiety. And an earlier analysis of the Alameda County group (this one expanded to include 5,200 people) found those attending a religious service at least weekly had a 25 percent lower mortality rate than infrequent attendees.

Researchers have also found a correlation between religious attendance and immune function. A University of Iowa study of 557 older adults reported that regular churchgoers were 65 percent less likely to have elevated levels of interleukin-6, an immune system marker for inflammation and cardiovascular disease.

Hummer says scientists are investigating several mechanisms that may explain this remarkable survival advantage. "Most religious groups teach individuals to take care of their bodies and minds," he says, pointing to teachings advocating less alcohol use and smoking avoidance. A 2004 study found that churchgoers ate 25 percent more fruits and vegetables, and largely the ones delivering the biggest nutritional punch, like broccoli, citrus fruits, carrots, and dark leafy vegetables. The study authors says the findings suggest that healthful habits taught at church were taking hold. Churches, temples and mosques also provide a type of social support hard to find with a bowling league or Rotary Club. Congregation members often give each other support that goes beyond the occasional favor. Members in need, such the homebound, may receive regular food deliveries, rides to the doctor, and abundant advice.

But beyond practical matters, regular religious attendees often experience a heightened sense of well being, confident they can turn to a divine source of power. "It could be that people really are more at ease in life, with taking on difficulties in life, with turning over their problems to a higher power," Hummer says. A few scientists have even speculated that the effect could be due to divine intervention, but Hummer isn't among them. "I'd be really hard-pressed to point to something like that. I guess I'm more of a pragmatist."

Making It Real

Most scientists aren't pursuing this line of research to encourage more religious service attendance. But they readily state that if you are regularly attending, it appears you're giving yourself an important health advantage.

Researchers emphasize that actually attending service, not simply practicing a faith at home, has the strongest health effect, likely due to the nature of the social support found in churches, synagogues, and mosques. Religious organizations provide a type of health-boosting support almost impossible to find elsewhere. "One of the things that might be different with religious involvement is this doctrine of how to live your life and the concern for others in the community," Hummer notes.

For those not religiously inclined, these findings on religion and health may still provide valuable insights.

The results underscore the health implications of social connections. They also reveal that the quality of the connections matter as much as the quantity. The more supportive the group, the greater sense you have of being able to rely upon its members in time of need. The findings also point to the benefit of reducing sources of stress, either by avoiding them or by adopting a different perspective on problems and challenges.

To Learn More

For additional information on the relationship between religion or spirituality and health, including links to journal articles, visit Duke University's Center for Spirituality, Theology and Health at www.dukespiritualityandhealth.org.

CHAPTER 39

Live with Purpose

In Japan, a movement is afoot to spread the practice of *ikigai*, which in Western parlance roughly means raison d'être, or reason for living. But the word in Japanese transcends the meaning of the French phrase. *Ikigai* means a way of living, one that fosters the development of a positive purpose in life and a sense of enthusiasm and satisfaction.

It's a philosophy widely known in Japan. And, as Japanese society ages, the government is promoting *ikigai* among older Japanese to encourage their independence and relieve the burdens on families and social support systems in caring for them. The *Ikigai* Foundation in Japan even provides advisors to help seniors live more productive, healthful lives. And with increasingly positive views of the aging process, similar movements are arising in other countries.

However, as the Japanese have found, discovering a renewed sense of purpose can be daunting, particularly for people who once devoted their lives to family and work. The goal sounds loftier than many people can envision achieving. Who can hope to approach the contributions to humanity of preeminent figures like Nelson Mandela, Mother Teresa, and Jimmy Carter?

But as Walter M. Bortz, MD, a leading authority on successful aging and author of the bestselling book, *Dare to Be 100*, notes, you can find purpose and meaning in small efforts. "Do my plants need me, does my dog need me to take him for a walk? It need not have high value in terms of prestige," he says. One could also join worthy causes, become immersed in valuable research, or make an art of writing letters to the editor, he adds. The list is endless.

What Scientists Know

The influence of cultivating a sense of purpose in life on health and longevity has been well researched in Japan. A study of more than 1,000 older Japanese found that those practicing *ikigai* lived significantly longer than their non-practicing counterparts. Another study involving male students reported that "those who had strong motivation for achievement of a purpose were significantly less depressed than those who had no motivation." Researchers also found varying reasons for people to adopt *ikigai*. A study of elderly Japanese reports that those in rural areas were more inclined to practice it when they had strong family structures, while their urban counterparts were more likely to adopt *ikigai* after a crisis such as a hospitalization.

Researchers in other countries have come to similar conclusions about the influence of a sense of purpose in promoting mental and physical health. One Danish study correlates finding a meaning in life with "becoming well again." A Finnish study found elders with the highest cognitive functioning had retained a sense of purpose. These high-functioning women and men were also more likely to volunteer in their free time. And Michigan researchers found that it's never too late to instill a sense of purpose into day-to-day life. The researchers discovered that older men and women taught basic principles about achieving quality of life soon cultivated a greater sense of meaning about their lives. These elders later fared better in health than even those with strong social support, the latter long viewed as one of the best predictors of good health and longevity.

Making It Real

So what exactly is purpose in life? Viktor E. Frankl, author of the seminal 1946 work *Man's Search For Meaning*, wrote that peoples' "main concern consists in fulfilling a meaning and in actualizing values, rather than in the mere gratification and satisfaction of drives and instincts." Frankl survived internment in German concentration camps during World War II, and in the book chronicles how the horrors of the experience forged his core philosophy: humanity's primary motivating force is a search for purpose and meaning in life. In the camps, he realized that once a person "knows the 'why' for his existence, and will be able to bear almost any 'how.'" He became convinced that possessing a sense of purpose keeps people alive in the face of adversity. Frankl died in 1997 at the age of 92.

Cultivating a sense of purpose in life is often grounded in the concept of giving your talents for the good of others. This concept is rooted in one of the basic laws of nature, says Bortz. He believes that the laws of thermodynamics even govern human behavior. "For us to be born and just consume creates a thermal disequilibrium. The only way we can keep equilibrium is to keep putting energy back in. It's the organizing principle."

Bortz puts this philosophy into practice by adopting the belief that as he grows older, his degree of responsibility increases. It's an overarching tenet of his life. "The older we become, the more responsible we should be, because we have shaped the environment to our usage," he says. For Bortz, this means remaining engaged in the affairs of life, and in using his talents for a higher purpose. Now in his mid-seventies, Bortz says many people do the opposite as they age, pulling away with friends, family and their previous social circle.

He also counsels people to strive to experience "flow" in their work, in which one become so immersed in an endeavor that time passes by almost unnoticed. Bortz adds that, "not only does living this fully engaged life allow you to live longer and better, but it allows you to die quicker. You want to go with your foot fully on the accelerator. You don't want to go in idle."

To Learn More

Read Frankl's book, "Man's Search For Meaning." For a carefully researched overview of spirituality and purpose in life, visit talk show host Oprah Winfrey's website at www.oprah.com. Click on the "Spirit and Self" link on the home page.

CHAPTER 40

Get the Right Touch

In the 19th century, children in orphanages had poor odds for survival, regardless of how clean or well-fed they were kept. More than half of infants in orphanages died in their first year, writes Ashley Montagu in his seminal work, *Touching: The Human Significance of the Skin*.

Many of these babies perished from what doctors called "marasmus," a Greek word that means "wasting away." Researchers investigating the tragic trend found that these deaths occurred most often in the "best" institutions, where conditions were kept as sterile as possible, and touching of infants was discouraged to prevent the spread of diseases.

Then in the late 1920s, a few prescient physicians instituted the practice of holding the babies in pediatric wards a few times a day. Within a year of adopting this protocol at Bellevue Hospital in New York, infant mortality rates fell more than threefold, to less than 10 percent, with the decline attributed to the physical contact.

Touch isn't a hot topic in mainstream medicine, but a number of studies—and intuition—make a convincing case that it matters in achieving wellness, for children and adults. In our touch-averse culture, it may be one of the most neglected aspects of maintaining health.

Yet the healing power of touch isn't a new concept is in medicine. The "laying on of hands" by ancient physicians was the most common form of treatment, according to Tiffany Field, PhD, in her book, *Touch*.

"I think touch is just as necessary to good health as diet and exercise," says Field, who's also the director of the Touch Research Institute at the University of Miami's School of Medicine.

Dean Ornish, MD, the bestselling author and director of the Preventive Medicine Research Institute, agrees. He says that touch is one of the pillars of wholesome living, and that "instead viewing these as luxuries of life, you can see them as essential as eating or breathing or sleeping."

People regularly receiving lots of touch report "that they don't have to go to the doctor as often," Field notes. "People always say they feel better and they're more content with their lives."

What Scientists Know

Humans, like many animals, possess a biological imperative to touch. While there's a deep yearning for physical contact, it's thwarted by our culture's strict limits on touching.

That was aptly illustrated by the work of Sidney Jourard, a researcher who traveled the world to watch how often couples touched one another in cafes.

In Puerto Rico, he saw that couples touched each other 180 times an hour, while in expressive France, they touched on average 110 times in an hour. But in the United States, it was a mere two times per hour, and in staid London, couples didn't touch each other once in an hour!

Skin, the body's largest organ, is rich with receptors sensitive to heat, cold, touch, and pain. Stimulation of these receptors, which give us a silent but powerful connection with the outside world, is vital to health.

A study of women with breast cancer found that regular massage reduces depression and anxiety and enhances dopamine and serotonin levels. It also boosts levels of lymphocytes and natural killer cells, which are white blood cells that, among other functions, clear out cancer cells and viruses from the body. Research on young men with HIV found a similar immune system response to massage.

Recent research has discovered that massage results in a significant decrease in heart rate and blood pressure. Massage also reduces cortisol levels, one of the primary stress hormones that can lower immunity, damage brain cells, and promote heart disease.

Research from the Touch Research Institute and other academic centers also show that therapies like massage or stroking reduce blood glucose levels in diabetics, alleviate depression, and stimulate heightened awareness.

Making It Real

To gently move beyond cultural limitations on touching, Ornish, in his book *Love & Survival: The Scientific Basis for the Healing Power of Intimacy*, advises simple steps like giving people a pat on the back or "a hug when they've done a good job—or even when they haven't." Shake hands more often with colleagues, he suggests, and "hold hands with your beloved."

Field describes imaginative, but socially sanctioned, ways to increase healthy physical contact with people. Take up dancing, or start playing a sport that involves lots of physical contact. Give friends and families more massages. The person giving the massage also experiences the benefits of touch, studies show. Get massages, manicures and pedicures for yourself. It's moderate pressure that provides the best kind of touch, says Field, so even steps like bathing oneself with a loofah sponge or using a natural hairbrush provide healthy stimulation. And don't forget our furry friends. Owning a pet is a terrific way to integrate more connection and touch into your life.

The first step, Ornish says, is just being aware of the value of physical contact. "When we understand the healing power of touching, we can look for ways of increasing our contact with other people, while respecting their boundaries."

To Learn More

Visit the Touch Research Institute's website at www.miami.edu/touch-research.

CHAPTER 41

Heed Your Homocysteine

In 1968, when Kilmer McCully, MD, made a fortuitous observation about an obscure genetic disease, he never could have imagined that it would change our understanding of heart disease, and in the process derail his career. While reviewing the cases of two children with the rare disease homocystinuria, the Harvard researcher noticed that both children died with advanced cardiovascular disease. Homocystinuria arises out of the body's inability to break down the amino acid homocysteine. As a result, extremely high levels accumulate in the blood. In 1969, McCully proposed a radical idea—the children's damaged arteries weren't just a coincidence, but rather a direct result of the extreme levels of homocysteine. Perhaps, he suggested, even mildly elevated levels may pose a heart hazard to adults.

His homocysteine hypothesis came during the ascendancy of the cholesterol theory of cardiovascular disease, and it was met with indifference, skepticism and occasionally hostility. Over the next several years, McCully's hypothesis failed to gain acceptance, which eventually led to his dismissal from Harvard. Time, however, vindicated McCully. In 1995, the 10 authors of a landmark study in the New England Journal of Medicine paid homage to McCully's work when they opened their article citing his observations 25 years earlier. Since then, hundreds of studies have been published confirming the link between homocysteine and incidence of heart disease and stroke. Some even suggest that homocysteine levels are a more significant risk factor for cardiovascular disease than cholesterol. Recent research shows that homocysteine influence the development of numerous other diseases, such as cancer, osteoporosis, depression, and Alzheimer's disease. High homocysteine levels occur throughout the elderly population in the U.S., according to studies.

What Scientists Know

Homocysteine, a by-product of the breakdown of animal protein, is an amino acid found in the blood that's important for normal metabolism. The body maintains safe levels of homocysteine by converting excess amounts to a beneficial amino acid; folic acid and vitamins B6 and B12 play an essential role in this process. However, this conversion system lags when there's a shortage of these nutrients, and homocysteine levels become dangerously elevated. Chronically high homocysteine concentrations damage the lining of artery walls, causing them to become thickened, inelastic, and lined with plaque. Over time, this condition can lead to a heart attack or stroke. Researchers have found that there is a linear relationship between risk of heart disease and progressively higher levels of homocysteine. One study found that for each 3 mmol/L increase in homocysteine, there was a 35 percent increase in heart attack risk.

Scientists have recently discovered a convincing correlation between high homocysteine and dementia. In a 2003 study in *Lancet*, researchers found that elevated homocysteine was linked to brain cell death and the onset of Alzheimer's disease and other types of dementia. These scientists expressed the hope that reducing homocysteine levels with folic acid supplementation could significantly lower the incidence of these brain diseases. A *New England Journal of Medicine* study concluded that "an increased plasma homocysteine level is a strong, independent risk factor for the development of dementia and Alzheimer's disease."

Recent studies now suggest a connection between elevated homocysteine and certain cancers, including leukemia and breast cancer. High homocysteine levels appear to boost the rates of hip fractures. Those with the highest blood concentrations were up to four times more likely to break a hip than those with the lowest, according to a 2004 study. Researchers postulate that homocysteine may interfere with normal bone formation.

The amino acid is also linked with depression. In a study of nearly 6000 Norwegians, researchers found that those with the highest levels of homocysteine were nearly twice as likely to suffer from depression as those with the lowest.

Making It Real

The research is clear; it's important to know your homocysteine status. Whenever you are taking a blood test, insist that homocysteine be measured as well. It may not be covered by insurance, but it's worth the cost. Although some commercial labs suggest that a normal level can range between 5 mmol/L to 15 mmol/L, the risk of heart attack can vary four-fold between the extremes, according to studies. Any reading greater than 9 mmol/L should be a call to action.

Homocysteine levels can generally be controlled through supplementation with folic acid and vitamins B6 and B12. As a minimal precaution, take a multiple vitamin with 400 mcg of folic acid, and at least 3 mg of vitamin B6 and 5 mcg to 15 mcg of B12. Folate, the natural form of folic acid, is prevalent in green leafy vegetables, beans, and oranges, although it's not as bioavailable as the synthetic version found in supplements. Broccoli and bananas contain high levels of B6. And B12 is primarily found in red meats and egg yolks.

Be sure to check to your homocysteine concentrations regularly, as levels sometimes even remain elevated, despite supplementation. If you consume alcohol, even in moderation, be aware that alcohol inhibits the absorption of folic acid and B vitamins. Make sure to take extra supplements after you've been drinking to make up for the loss. And there's yet another good reason to begin a regular exercise program, as preliminary research suggests it directly lowers homocysteine levels.

To Learn More

Read McCully's 1997 book *The Homocysteine Revolution*. For developments on homocysteine levels and health, visit the National Institutes of Health's website at www.nih.gov, and type in "homocysteine" in the search box.

CHAPTER 42

Just Say "Om"

The meditative traditions like Buddhism and Hinduism have long made the case that humanity suffers from a kind of mass attention deficit disorder, and we're woefully ignorant of our compromised state. Few people can finish a page of reading without their mind wandering, a scattered state we regard as normal. Meditation, or mindfulness, which teaches its practitioners to train their minds to remain in the present, acts as an antidote to humanity's seemingly hardwired tendency to ricochet from thought to thought.

Meditation isn't just in the domain of Eastern cultures. Mark Abramson, MD, a dental surgeon who teaches meditation at Stanford University's School of Medicine, says it's a universal practice. Jesus Christ went to the desert to meditate, Abramson points out. Native American cultures practiced forms of meditation. It's by no means solely linked to spiritual pursuits; it's also practiced for non-secular reasons, such as stress reduction. "Our default setting is being stress laden," says Abramson. Meditation entails "teaching yourself to be calmly focused on what is actually happening right now," rather than worrying about real or anticipated problems.

Decades after the Beatles popularized meditation in Western culture through their training with Maharishi Mahesh Yogi, meditation has gone mainstream. About 10 million Americans now practice it, and hundreds of studies show they're protecting their health while improving their outlook.

What Scientists Know

The simple act of focusing thoughts inward and on the present has profound physiological and psychological effects. "As we focus our attention back to ourselves, we create an internal change that is very real physically," says Abramson.

Meditation has a striking effect on cardiovascular functioning. One of the early U.S. meditation researchers, Herbert Benson, MD, of Harvard Medical School, found that the meditators he studied on average slowed their heart rates 3 beats per minute and used 17 percent less oxygen while meditating. It's well-documented that blood pressure declines with meditation. A 2004 study found people with hypertension who meditated twice a day for four months had an average 3.5 point drop in blood pressure readings, while non-meditators experienced little or no decline. Yale University researchers also report that people with cardiovascular disease who began practicing meditation and yoga improved their artery dilation—an important indicator of cardiovascular health—by more than two thirds. A study in India found that short-term and long-term meditators had significantly lower blood pressure readings and cholesterol levels than non-meditators, even though all study participants maintained similar levels of physical activity.

Meditation also has a powerful influence in easing chronic stress. A recent study found that meditators shifted brain wave patterns to a more relaxing state and were less likely to experience a "fight or flight" response to stressors. Chronic triggering of this response is linked to the onset of many health conditions, such as cardiovascular disease, cancer, diabetes, and cognitive decline. Meditation's role in stress reduction may also aid cancer patients, one study concluded.

Immune function is bolstered in meditators, according to recent research. The calmer state of mind enjoyed by meditators was linked to significant increases in influenza antibodies following a flu vaccine injection—indicating the meditators' immune systems responded more robustly to the vaccination.

Meditation may affect cancer growth, according to preliminary findings. A recent study suggested that increases in levels of PSA—blood molecules linked with prostate cancer—slowed dramatically in men diagnosed with prostate cancer who began meditating and adhering to a low-saturated fat, high-fiber, plant-based diet. In three of the men, PSA rates actually declined.

Studies with fibromyalgia patients showed meditation reduced chronic pain, and earlier research linked it to the relief of chronic pain for a number of conditions. Meditation had a significant effect in curbing anxiety attacks, according to a three-year trial. One intriguing study tested the effect of meditation in clearing the painful rashes of psoriasis patients who were subject to a stressful treatment in a hot chamber with ultraviolet light. Those practicing meditation to ease the stress cleared up their skin at four times the rate of those who didn't meditate.

Making It Real

There are as many ways to meditate as there are cultures that practice it. Transcendental meditation teaches you to focus your mind by repeating a mantra for 15 to 20 minutes, while gently pushing aside other intruding thoughts. Other methods instruct you to focus on your breathing, or a pleasant image. The website listed below describes several easy meditation techniques, as do numerous books and tapes.

Abramson teaches not only sitting meditation, but a form of calming mindfulness one can maintain while active, such as during exercise. "You can make that a time to focus on the feelings of your body, rather than reading a newspaper or watching a television show as you're on the exercise bike. If you're a runner, you feel yourself running, you feel yourself breathing, you feel the air in your face, and that becomes meditation." Even that active form of mindfulness has physiological stress-reducing effects, he says.

However, the sitting meditations—which only require a comfortable chair, not the flexibility to sit lotus style—have a profound effect in helping you access your true emotions and values, he says. "For some people, sitting still brings them to a state that they're not used to. And that can be very good for you. It can reveal agitation and a lack of stillness in your life" that can be remedied.

To Learn More

For a comprehensive overview of the philosophy behind meditation, as well as various ways to practice it, visit www.how-to-meditate.org. This noncommercial site focuses on Buddhist meditation practices, although it's geared for a general audience.

CHAPTER 43

Visit Mother Nature

Listening to a chorus of birds, meandering alongside a sparkling creek, and reveling in the view of a crimson sunset are experiences that not only revive the soul, but restore health as well.

Enterprising scientists are exploring the connections between nature and health, and finding even brief encounters with the natural world reduce stress, speed healing and ease pain. Forays into wilderness areas or just relaxing in the town park also promote closeness among friends, families and spouses, increasing the strength of social connections, one of the most powerful influences on good health.

Experiences with nature effect health by providing a spiritually and psychologically calming experience, says Sara Warber, MD, author of a study called "Greening Healthcare," and the codirector of the Complementary and Alternative Medicine Research Center at the University of Michigan. "When you affect both those things positively, that also affects the body's ability to heal," she says.

The work of Warber and like-minded scientists occupies an obscure corner of the complementary medicine movement. But as the growing number of "healing gardens" in hospitals attest, their work is emerging from the shadows and into the light as studies show that time spent enjoying flowers, trees, birds, and sun can sometimes work better than medicine in improving health. And Warber emphasizes that nature can be found virtually anywhere you look—from the grandest vista to a scenic drive, or even in a simple potted plant.

"You don't have to be in the Grand Tetons to experience nature. Nature is all around us," she says. "That's one of our interests here, what we call nearby nature. Our goal is to make that more explicitly connected to health."

What Scientists Know

Nature can disarm killers like hypertension and chronic stress. In one study, participants were shown videos of work-related accidents to induce stress. They were then shown one of three video scenes: a natural area, urban traffic, or a pedestrian mall. Tests of muscle tension and blood pressure showed that those viewing the nature images recovered more quickly from stress than participants viewing the traffic or pedestrian scenes.

Field research found that after performing a demanding task, blood pressure levels dropped more rapidly in people sitting in a room with a view of trees than in those sitting in a viewless room. Walking in a nature reserve also led to lowered blood pressure, compared to a group of people walking through an urban setting. Those on the nature walk also felt less anger and more positive emotions than those trekking through the urban jungle. Other research showed that people viewing simulated drives through nature scenes recovered faster from mildly stressful events than those watching a simulated drive through an urban setting. Scientists believe interactions with nature stimulate the parasympathetic system, the part of the nervous system that slows down heart rate and lowers levels of stress hormones like cortisol.

This "green medicine" movement can also save impressive amounts of health care dollars, research shows. Researchers looked at 9 years of data on people admitted to a hospital for gallbladder surgery, and reported that patients who had a view of trees, compared with patients with a view of a brick wall, left almost a day earlier—staying roughly 8 days instead of 9. Remarkably, patients with the window view also took only one strong pain pill for every 2.5 pills taken by those with no view. Instead, they relied on lower-strength medicines, like aspirin, consuming more than twice the number of the milder, less costly pills as the patients viewing the brick wall. "That makes sense, because when people are anxious they feel more pain," says Warber. "So this is a great example of where addressing the more subtle aspects of the patient has effects in the physical body."

Even images of nature have a soothing effect. Patients in beds with curtains painted with nature scenes and surrounded by natural sounds experienced less pain after an operation than those without the natural enhancements.

Nature also helps restore a cognitive state called directed attention—in essence, concentration. Over time, the ability to concentrate on one task while suppressing your attention from others falters from fatigue. To restore directed attention, people need to take a break and become involved with "involuntary attention," in which the mind is drawn to whatever stimulates and attracts it, such as wild animals, attractive plants or lovely vistas.

Making It Real

It's extraordinarily simple to bring nature closer to your life, Warber says. Even a computer screensaver of an outdoors scene has a soothing effect. Add wilderness photos to your office and bring in plants. Put a birdfeeder or small garden outside your window. When you're driving, take a moment to enjoy the beauty of the trees lining the road. Walks in the wilderness are restorative, as are strolls through local parks. Sounds of nature are soothing; get a CD of bird songs or ocean waves, or purchase a small water fountain.

You can use the knowledge of nature's calming influence to buffer you from stress and even increase your capacity to respond to trying situations. "You have something you can do to protect yourself from stress," Warber says. "Practices that put you into this restful, relaxed, connected place help create a more resilient body that can respond when it is stressed." By lowering your overall stress level, she explains, you retain greater physiological capacity to rise to the challenge when true emergencies strike, rather than wearing your system down by remaining in an unnecessary state of alert.

To Learn More

The website of Bedscapes, a firm that markets products that use images of nature in hospital settings, has a section dedicated to research on the effect of nature on health. Visit the site at www.bedscapes.com and select the "Research Results" icon on the home page.

CHAPTER 44

Win an Oscar

There's another reason for actors clutch their newly won Oscars so tightly. That 13-inch gold statuette can actually add years to your life, an intriguing study recently reported.

Movie stars who have won an Oscar live on average four years longer than stars nominated but not selected. The longevity benefits appeared to accrue with additional wins; those winning multiple Oscars lived on average six years longer. Katherine Hepburn, who won a record four Oscars, lived to age 96. Anthony Quinn, the winner of two Academy Awards, lived to age 86, and George Burns, winner of one, famously made it to age 100. But Richard Burton, who was nominated seven times for an Academy Award but never won the prize, died at age 58.

The Oscar study is among the latest chapter in a volume of research linking social status and self-esteem to longevity. A recent survey found that Nobel prize-winning scientists who were members of the prestigious National Academy of Sciences lived an average of four years longer than Academy scientists who had never won the distinguished prize. One of the largest studies on social status and mortality—involving more than 10,000 British white-collar workers—found a direct correlation between higher job status and lowered risk of heart disease. Other research found that executives and managers enjoyed a longer life span than those in mid-level management, while blue-collar workers had the shortest lives.

While medical researchers have long known that low socioeconomic status predisposes people to health problems and shortened life spans, it was usually attributed to factors like limited access to health care and poor diets. But this recent crop of studies suggests something else is at work, since famous actors, accomplished scientists, and white collar workers have similar access to quality health care and certainly have incomes sufficient to ensure adequate diets.

What Scientists Know

University of Toronto researchers who embarked on their study of Academy Award winners realized this unique group could provide a fresh look at the phenomenon of social status and its link to increased longevity. This already advantaged group of actors were near the top of society's ladder. In addition, the Academy Awards show is one of the most widely shared experiences worldwide—it's beamed to more than 100 countries and draws an estimated one billion viewers. The evening's winners experience an unprecedented level of acclaim. In contrast, most studies on social status have compared disadvantaged workers with more privileged ones.

The researchers recorded the life spans of all those ever nominated for an Academy Award for leading and supporting acting roles. They also created a control group of performers who had never been nominated, but had appeared in the same films for which the Academy Award winners had won their prize. The scientists found that winning the gold statuette conferred a four-year survival advantage compared to those nominated but not selected, an advantage that increased to six years for those winning two or more Oscars. Those earning a nomination—itself a high honor—actually had about the same life span as actors who were never nominated.

Donald Redelmeier, MD, one of the scientists conducting the study, which was published in the *Annals of Internal Medicine*, says the findings suggest that the enhanced self-esteem imparted by winning a prestigious award exerts a powerful effect in improving health, even in those with every advantage in life. "Once you've got a major accomplishment that nobody can take away from you, that gives you a sense of self-esteem and makes you much more resilient to all of the other stressors in life," he says in a radio interview. That, in turn, could lower levels of stress hormones linked to cardiovascular disease and other health problems, as well improve immune system function. He also writes in the study that newly prominent Oscar winners are more likely to "preserve their image by continually avoiding disgraceful behaviors and maintaining exemplary conduct." In contrast, another study notes that low self-esteem is linked to depression, which leaves people vulnerable to a variety of ailments. Lowered self-esteem can also reduce motivation to maintain good health behaviors.

The study of British white collar workers found that mortality rates were three times worse in the workers in the lowest job grade than those in the highest grade, and this was after accounting for factors like smoking habits, blood pressure, and cholesterol levels. The scientists running the study concluded that the lower-grade occupations were associated with a lack of control over work, greater work pressures, and less social support outside of work, all factors linked to poorer health.

Making It Real

Obviously, few people will ever win an Oscar and have a chance to garner its life-extending benefits. But as bioethicist Arthur Caplan, PhD, states, the Oscar study "does at least suggest that money isn't everything in life. Achievement and social recognition count too."

But getting to the top of the heap—for example, earning a salesperson of the year award, acing an exam, or winning a local competition—can instill some of the same self-esteem boosts enjoyed by winners of any magnitude. Achievement also promotes positive thinking, another attribute strongly linked to lowered stress and the practice of protective health behaviors.

You can use knowledge of self-esteem's link to health to boost other people's well being, as well. As Caplan writes, "Parents, teachers, politicians, and the media who have the power to honor and acknowledge social worth might keep this in mind."

To Learn More

Read *The Six Pillars of Self-Esteem* by psychologist Nathaniel Branden, one of the world's authorities on self-esteem. For more information on his work on building self-esteem, visit www.nathanielbranden.com.

CHAPTER 45

Look on the Bright Side

Decades ago, researchers noticed that animals facing adverse events from which they couldn't escape developed weakened immune systems. In the 1970s, scientists turned their attention to humans to investigate how a similar sense of helplessness in the face of adversity affected health. Attitudes of optimism and pessimism, they found, were major determinants in who persevered through challenges, and who succumbed to helpless feelings.

Medical researchers and doctors widely agree that optimistic patients, on the whole, fare better when undergoing medical treatments—either by experiencing better outcomes or maintaining a better quality of life while contending with illness. Numerous studies also show the protective effect of optimism in preventing chronic stress and strengthening the immune system. Conversely, pessimistic outlooks are strikingly correlated with poorer health outcomes and earlier death.

Martin Seligman, PhD, a leading researcher on optimism and health, and author of *Learned Optimism: How to Change Your Mind and Your Life*, describes pessimistic people as those who interpret negative events as permanent and pervasive. Optimistic people, on the other hand, view adverse events as temporary, controllable, and confined to one area of life.

Robert C. Colligan, PhD, a researcher with the Mayo Clinic who helped design a standard personality test now used to assess levels of optimism and pessimism, notes that Seligman's theories also predict that those identified as pessimists "are at increased risk for later problems with achievement in school and in their career, with their physical health and with emotional stress, particularly depression."

Research over the past 30 years, Colligan notes, supports Seligman's predictions.

What Scientists Know

In a recent study on optimism, researchers assessed attitudes in a group of more than 900 Canadians aged 65 to 85. The participants were asked their responses to statements like, "I still have many goals to strive for," and "I often feel that life is full of promise." Nine years later, 42 percent of the group had died, and in a 2004 article, study researchers reported that those rated "highly optimistic" were 55 percent less likely to have died than those with the most negative outlook. The optimists also had a 23 percent reduction in mortality from heart disease, even after taking into account their health history.

In explaining possibilities for the disparities, the scientists says that pessimists may be more likely to smoke and to have high blood pressure and excess weight, and they may be less likely to follow to guidelines for improving health. Or it may be that a hopeful, cheerful outlook provides biological boosts for a stronger immune system.

One study of 90 first-year law students found such a correlation between optimism and immune system function. Suzanne Segerstrom, PhD, a researcher who has extensively studied the effects of optimism on immunity, reported that the students at the start of the school year showed similar levels of immune system function, regardless of whether they were pessimistic or optimistic about the rigors of the upcoming year. However, by mid-year, the optimists had more of the powerful helper T cells, which amplify immune system responses. The T cells showed higher cytotoxicity, or ability to kill cancer cells in lab tests. Segerstrom says the changes in immune system function could be attributable to two characteristics of optimists: they find challenging events less stressful than do pessimists, and they experience negative moods like anxiety and depression less frequently.

An oft-cited 30-year study from the Mayo Clinic, which Colligan coauthored, found that those assessed as pessimistic at the start of the study had a 19 percent higher death rate. Earlier research on patients undergoing heart surgery notes those with an optimistic outlook had a faster recovery while hospitalized and returned to normal activities more quickly.

In deference to skeptics of research on optimism and health, some studies have also shown that a positive outlook had no effect on outcomes with serious illnesses like cancer. And these patients may feel doubly dejected, some researchers note, as though they simply weren't "positive enough" to beat their disease. But scientists on both side of the optimism/health aisle generally that agree a positive perspective can't hurt, as long as it doesn't impose guilt if a disease still gets the upper hand. At minimum, an optimistic outlook can improve the experience of life when faced with a grave disease. As Colligan states, "It is equally important to think about quality of life, and not just life span."

Making It Real

Optimism needs to be combined with action for real results, scientists emphasize. It's the motivation fueled by an optimistic disposition that encourages people to maintain healthful lifestyles and adopt outlooks that circumvent stressful responses to challenges or crisis. As Seligman states, "Casual reading of the popular literature on health and optimism might lead one to conclude that good health is all in a person's mind." However, he continues, "behavior is the critical link; behavior must have a realistic link to health."

Optimism can also be viewed as developing a positive resilience in life. The American Psychological Association, in its online primer, "10 Ways to Build Resilience," counsels people to cultivate a healthier outlook by building good relationships, refusing to see crises as insurmountable, accepting that change is a part of life, continually moving toward goals, taking decisive action, looking for opportunities for self-discovery, nurturing a positive view of yourself, and keeping events in perspective.

To Learn More

Read *Learned Optimism: How to Change Your Mind and Your Life* by Martin Seligman. Visit the American Psychological Association's public support website at http://helping.apa.org and type in "Resilience" in the search box.

CHAPTER 46

Choose Your Fats Wisely

The American public can be forgiven its confusion about fat in the diet. No sooner did health officials declare war on fat, particularly saturated fats, than Robert Atkins, MD, in 1972 released his bestselling book touting the virtues of a high-fat diet to lose weight painlessly. Atkins' reign was eclipsed briefly by the Pritikin and Ornish diet plans that cut fat to the bone, only to have sand kicked in their faces by the South Beach Diet, essentially a modified Atkins.

Until recently, the role of fat in our body has been poorly understood. Once regarded as simply an easily stored energy source, today we have a far more sophisticated understanding of fat's function in normal metabolism. Dietary fat provides the raw material for cell membranes, hormones, and the insulation that surrounds nerves. Fats help regulate blood clotting and muscle contraction. Our brains are largely made of fat. We now know that eating good fats, among other health benefits, can prevent cardiovascular disease and reduce the likelihood of Alzheimer's disease, diabetes, and macular degeneration. Dietary fats even transport vital nutrients like carotenoids and vitamins A, E, D, and K from the intestine to the bloodstream. In his book, *Eat, Drink, and Be Healthy*, Walter Willett, MD, of the Harvard School of Public Health states, "Eating more good fats—staying away from bad ones—is second only to weight control on the list of healthy nutritional strategies."

What Scientists Know

Fats fall into four basic categories: saturated, like those in red meat or dairy; monounsaturated, like olive oil; polyunsaturated, such as corn oil; and trans-fats, found in commercial products like Crisco. Saturated and trans-fats are solid at room temperature, while monounsaturated and polyunsaturated fats, usually referred to as oils, are liquid. The body can actually create most of the fats it needs, either by converting dietary fats or synthesizing them from carbohydrates. But some are obtained only from dietary sources, and thus are called essential fats.

Saturated fats are primarily found in meat, dairy foods, and a few plant-based foods, such as coconuts. It's debatable if we need to eat any saturated fats at all, as the body can manufacture what it needs. What is agreed upon is that dietary saturated fats boost cholesterol levels, increase blood fats, and promote unnecessary blood clotting—all risk factors for cardiovascular disease.

Trans-fats were created when scientists heated vegetable oil, together with the catalyst nickel, and produced a strange fat that was semi-solid at room temperature. It was also easy to store and resistant to rancidity. Without this breakthrough, we wouldn't have margarine or Crisco. But we'd also have 30,000 fewer deaths from heart disease, according to Harvard's Willett. In 2002, the Institute of Medicine reported that there are no safe levels of trans-fatty acid consumption. They raise levels of LDL cholesterol, lower the "good" HDL variety, and increase levels of triglycerides. Some studies also link them to cancer and increased rates of diabetes.

Monounsaturated fats are found in oils such as olive, peanut, and canola, and a few foods, like avocados and nuts. They are the fats of choice in the "heart healthy" Mediterranean diet. In this diet, olive oil is a staple, while butter and other dairy products, as well as red meat, are consumed sparingly.

Polyunsaturated fats are generally regarded as heart healthy, and studies show they improve the ratio of HDL to LDL cholesterol and modulate levels of triglycerides. Our bodies don't make polyunsaturated fats, so we get these essential fats from plant foods like corn, soybeans, seeds, nuts, and whole grains, and from fatty fish like salmon and sardines. Polyunsaturated fats include the omega-6 and, to a lesser extent, omega-3 fat groups.

In recent years, the omega-3s have generated considerable excitement for their myriad health benefits.

Innumerable studies have shown that omega-3 fats reduce inflammation, decrease heart arrhythmia, prevent clotting, lower total cholesterol levels, and moderate triglycerides in the blood. People eating just two to three servings of coldwater fish a week have significantly fewer heart attacks. A recent study in *Lancet* reported that people with heart disease consuming high levels of omega-3 fatty acids had far more stable arterial plaque than those with heart disease on typical Western diets. These fats also appear to prevent or reduce age-related cognitive impairment and may delay the onset of Alzheimer's disease.

Making It Real

Find the good fats. Use olive oil on salads and for cooking. Eat fish two to three times a week, particularly wild salmon. When fresh wild salmon isn't available, try the canned variety. If you're not a fan of fish, consider a fish oil supplement from a reputable manufacturer. Flaxseed meal is an excellent source of omega-3 fatty acids. It has a nutty flavor that works well on cereals and salads.

Eat more nuts, such as pecans, almonds, walnuts, and peanuts. Not only do they provide essential fats, but they're high in protein, vitamins, and minerals. Instead of snacks such as potato chips and cheese puffs, you can enjoy a snack of nuts for roughly the same number of calories. And eggs are an excellent source of beneficial fats, and are low in calories and high in protein and several vitamins.

Devise ways to cut back on saturated fats, such as those found in cheese, whole-milk dairy products, and red meat. Eliminate trans-fatty acids, which are also called hydrogenated fats on food labels. They are often hidden in commercial baked and fried goods.

Because fat is necessary for the absorption of many of the micronutrients in fruits and vegetables, particularly the carotenoids and the fat-soluble vitamins, it's a good idea to eat fruits and vegetables in a meal with fat sources such as fish, salad dressings, and avocados.

To Learn More

Visit the Harvard School of Public Health's website at www.hsph.harvard.edu/nutritionsource and select the "Fats & Cholesterol" icon.

CHAPTER 47

Mine for Minerals

Minerals don't get nearly the attention they deserve. Yet without them, our muscles wouldn't move, our heart wouldn't beat, and our bones would collapse. Minerals play essential roles in the creation of proteins, bones, countless enzymes, and hormones, and act as electrical conductors throughout the body.

Minerals are elements derived from the Earth's crust, and enter the food chain when plants absorb them. We ingest them directly from plants or indirectly through animal-based foods. We consume 60 or so minerals—22 of which are considered essential—and they comprise four percent of our body weight. They include such notables as calcium, potassium, magnesium, sodium, zinc, and iron. Among the lesser-known minerals are chromium, boron, copper, and selenium.

Optimal blood levels of minerals, studies show, help prevent several forms of cancer, reduce the incidence of heart attacks and strokes, bolster the immune system and help regulate cholesterol levels. They've also been linked to lower rates of diabetes, hypertension, and osteoporosis. However, just like certain vitamins, while optimal levels promote health, amounts in the extreme can be toxic.

These elements are classified as either macro or trace minerals, depending upon the widely varying quantities the body needs. For instance, the recommended daily intake of potassium is 70,000 times that of selenium, yet both are essential to good health.

What Scientists Know

Magnesium participates in more than 300 metabolic processes, including the vital function of converting carbohydrates and fats into energy. Synthesis of DNA, RNA, and proteins depend on magnesium, and it's involved in virtually all hormonal reactions. Magnesium plays a direct role in muscle contraction, normal heart rhythm, and the transmission of nerve impulses. Deficiencies of this mineral can lead to hypertension, congestive heart failure, and heart attacks. People with diets high in magnesium have 50 percent fewer heart attacks and strokes than those consuming the least amount. Recent studies show that magnesium helps prevent the onset of diabetes.

Selenium, once thought to be toxic and even carcinogenic, received a clean bill of health from the government in 1979, when it declared selenium an essential mineral. Selenium is a vital component of glutathione, one of the most potent antioxidants that the body manufactures. Studies show that selenium helps prevent lung, colon, and prostate cancers. In a landmark study, more than 1,300 men took 200 mcg daily of selenium for 10 years. At the study's end, the selenium group had 46 percent fewer lung cancers, 58 percent fewer colon cancers, and a remarkable 63 percent lower rate of prostate cancer, compared to the placebo group. Selenium also boosts the immune system, studies show. It supports the function of "killer" T cells and appears to slow the progression of viral diseases like influenza and hepatitis B and C.

Potassium is so important to human health that the Institute of Medicine in 2004 increased its recommended daily intake from 3,500 mg to 4,700 mg. Potassium facilitates the electrochemical impulses that control the firing of nerve cells, and it plays a crucial role in the regulation of blood pressure. The mineral also slows the onset of cardiovascular disease. A recent study of more than 43,000 men showed that those with the highest level of daily potassium intake, 4,300 mg, were 38 percent less likely to suffer a stroke than those consuming the least. One widely cited study found that a 400 mg daily increase in potassium intake—the amount found in one banana—decreased stroke incidence by 40 percent. Potassium helps preserve bone density, and deficiencies may lead to hypertension, depression, muscle weakness, slow reflexes, and fatigue.

Calcium is the most abundant mineral in the body, with 99 percent bound in bone and teeth. The remaining one percent floats in extracellular fluids, facilitating functions like nerve cell transmissions, muscle contractions, and hormonal secretions. Calcium's role in bone health is well known, but the complexity of its relationships with other nutrients isn't. The United States has among the highest intakes of calcium worldwide, yet we also have one of the highest rates of osteoporosis. Numerous studies conclude that the prevention of osteoporosis depends upon much more than calcium alone. Bone health can't be maintained in the absence of weight-bearing activities and adequate levels of micronutrients like vitamin D, magnesium, and potassium.

Making It Real

Magnesium deficiency is on the rise, due to the difficulty of consuming enough magnesium in the typical American diet. The government advises women to get 310 mg/day and men to get 400 mg/day. Consider a supplement, unless you eat generous amounts of nuts, beans, brown rice, wheat germ, whole wheat flour, oats, apples, bananas, and leafy green vegetables.

Most Americans get about half the potassium they need for optimal health, the Institute of Medicine states. Since extremely high levels of potassium can cause kidney and heart distress, don't take supplements without consulting a doctor. Most people can consume optimal levels with a diet abundant in fish, grains, fruits, and vegetables. Good sources of potassium include bananas, oranges, broccoli, spinach, and potatoes.

The average diet provides about 100 mcg of selenium a day, which exceeds the RDA of 70 mcg for men and 55 mcg for women. However, studies show selenium intakes of 200 mcg/day, even in people not overtly deficient, stimulate the immune system and may protect against certain cancers. Because of toxic side effects, do not exceed an intake of 400 mcg/day. Good sources include Brazil nuts, whole grains, seafood, chicken, pork, and beef. If you take a supplement, look for yeast-based selenium.

Calcium is available in scores of supplements, and good dietary sources include dairy products, spinach, broccoli, pinto beans, and red beans. It's essential to consume vitamin D, up to 1,000 mg/day, to maximize calcium absorption. Experts recommended consuming 1,000 mg/day of calcium for adults, and 1,200 mg/day for those 51 and older. Take no more than 500 mg at one time, since amounts beyond that generally can't be absorbed.

To Learn More

For a thorough discussion of the health effects and sources of minerals, visit the Linus Pauling Institute's Micronutrient Information Center's website at http://lpi.oregonstate.edu/infocenter/minerals.html.

CHAPTER 48

Get Out of the Hospital Alive

It's about the last thing on your mind when heading to the hospital: Will I die at the hands of the people hired to heal me?

It's a chilling thought. But a 1999 report that stunned the nation showed that prospect isn't so preposterous. The prestigious Institute of Medicine's astonishing report, "To Err is Human," describes how an estimated 44,000 to 98,000 people die annually in the United States because of errors by health care professionals. A 2004 study asserts that the IOM figures were actually low. reporting that 600,000 people died during the previous three years due to medical errors. The numbers triggered controversy, but if they're correct, that makes medical errors the 6th leading cause of death in the United States, more than cancers of prostate, breast, and colon combined.

Other medical experts contend that both reports understate the magnitude of the problem, citing a *Journal of the*

American Medical Association study showing that 106,000 patients die annually due to adverse drug reactions alone. And, whatever the actual number may be, add to the mix another estimated 88,000 patient fatalities from infections contracted in health care facilities, most of which are preventable. The situation prompted one researcher to say that the crisis is the equivalent of several jumbo jets crashing each week.

The belief that the American health care system is the best in the world is simply a myth, says Arthur Levin, MPH, the only public member of the IOM committee and the director of the Center for Medical Consumers in New York City. "I think one of the things that can be stricken from the rhetoric is that we have the best health care system in the world," he says. "The American health care system is simply failing to deliver safe and quality care."

The World Health Organization agrees. In 2004, it ranked the U.S. health care system 37th worldwide—between Costa Rica and Slovenia.

What Scientists Know

Seventeen-year-old Jesica Santillan died in 2003 after getting a heart-lung transplant from an incompatible donor at Duke University Medical Center. A health reporter for the Boston Globe, Betsy Lehman, died from an overdose of chemotherapy drugs. Ben Kolb, 8, died of a medication error while undergoing routine surgery.

Research points to numerous factors behind the tragedy of preventable medical errors: the nationwide nursing shortages, HMOs and insurance companies concerned with controlling costs, disjointed delivery of medical services, and health care managers' resistance to establishing quality control procedures or to purchasing electronic record-keeping systems. Even getting doctors to write legible prescriptions—a frequently cited problem—is often difficult.

As a result of the new spate of research on medical errors, some initiatives are under way to improve patient safety in hospitals. At Mercy Health Center in Oklahoma City, doctors cut infection rates by nearly 80 percent for major surgeries in 2003 after adopting federal guidelines for preventing such infections. A study by St. Paul and Marine Insurance Company showed that stress prevention programs in a 700-bed hospital, which included streamlining hospital procedures, resulted in a 50 percent decline in medication errors (and a 70 percent reduction in malpractice claims among 22 hospitals implementing the changes).

While these examples are encouraging, they're largely sporadic and the medical establishment and federal government still aren't responding with nearly the urgency the situation demands, Levin says. That means the onus, at this point, is on health care consumers to arm themselves with information and strategies to protect themselves from becoming an unfortunate statistic.

Making It Real

"It's a sad commentary that we can't guarantee that people are safe in the system," Levin says. "I mean, we don't ask people, before they get on the airlines, to go down with the copilot and check the tires and hydraulics and make sure that the plane is safe to fly." Until medical quality control enters the 21st century, there are a few things a patient can do.

First and foremost, educate yourself about your own medical condition before walking through the doors of a healthcare facility, Levin says. Don't be shy about asking questions of your health care provider.

Always bring someone to serve as your advocate during any major encounter in a health care setting, Levin says. "When you're not well, you may not be vigorous enough to protect yourself," he explains. Ask about all drugs being prescribed, and why, as well as potential adverse reactions with other drugs or supplements you're taking.

Get a second opinion when any significant surgery is proposed. If your doctor is offended, get another doctor. Second opinions are routine in medicine, and are frequently covered by insurance.

To protect yourself from hospital-acquired infections, insist that health workers, including doctors, wash their hands before examination. You'd be surprised how many health care workers skip this step, according to studies.

To Learn More

To view the federal Agency for Healthcare Research and Quality Patient fact sheet, "20 Tips to Help Prevent Medical Errors," visit www.ahrq.gov/consumer. You can also order the publication, free of charge, by calling (800) 358-9295.

To find out if your treatment plan is based on the latest scientific evidence, visit www.guideline.gov. It lists current treatment guidelines for most physical and mental conditions.

To learn how to prevent hospital-acquired infections, go to www.surgicalinfectionprevention.org.

CHAPTER 49

Don't Become a Statistic

During the first four decades of life, more people die of preventable injuries than any other cause. Over the course of a lifetime, accidents stand as the fifth leading cause of death among Americans, ahead of diabetes and influenza. In 2001, more than 100,000 people died from unintentional injuries, ranging from car accidents to falls or drownings, according to the Centers for Disease Control and Prevention.

Then there's the enormous toll from the crippling disabilities caused by accidents. The National Safety Council estimates that for every one person killed by an accident, another 54 sustain a disabling injury, one that oftentimes leads to premature death.

Safety experts say that roughly 90 percent of unintentional injuries are preventable. In a quest to lower these accident rates, the CDC and other health agencies have launched initiatives to teach accident prevention strategies and to urge the avoidance of risky behaviors. These measures include warnings about the dangers of driving while drowsy, the importance of installing carbon monoxide alarms along with smoke alarms, the hazards of biking without a helmet, and precautionary steps to avoid becoming a victim of a medication error.

What Scientists Know

Every year, more than 40,000 people die in automobile crashes in the United States. Nearly half of these fatalities are alcohol-related, and a least a third involve excess speed. Inattentiveness while driving, such as tending to small children or talking on a cell phone, accounts for about one quarter of vehicle crashes. Drivers falling asleep at the wheel causes at least 1,500 fatalities annually, according to the U.S. Department of Transportation, a figure that's almost certainly an underestimate, the agency added.

One out of every five vehicle occupants still doesn't regularly use a seatbelt, yet in a recent year almost two-thirds of vehicle occupants who were killed weren't wearing one. And safe driving extends to smart strategies for sharing the road. About 5,000 fatalities annually result from crashes between cars and big rigs, and 98 times out of 100, it's the car occupants that die, not the truck drivers. As most people can attest, road rage—in which aggressive drivers tailgate, weave in and out of traffic, yell, and gesticulate—is on the rise. The American Automobile

Association conservatively estimates that at least 12,000 accidents during a recent six-year period were caused by aggressive drivers.

Approximately 1,000 people a year die from bicycle injuries, and another 600,000 end up in emergency rooms. Wearing a bike helmet reduces the risk of serious injury by 85 percent, according to the U.S. Consumer Product Safety Commission. However, half of bike riders either never or infrequently wear a helmet.

Poisonings, the third leading cause of accidental deaths in the United States, caused more than 14,000 fatalities in 2001. Adverse drug reactions, overdoses of legal or illegal drugs, and carbon monoxide poisonings account for the majority of these fatalities. Carbon monoxide, a colorless and odorless gas which comes from combustion of fuels like propane or wood, enters enclosed spaces through leaks in fuel-burning appliances, or by using equipment designed for outdoor use, like grills or heaters, indoors.

Drownings caused more than 3,000 deaths in 2001. Up to half of drownings in adults and adolescents are linked to alcohol use. The lack of monitoring of swimmers is another leading factor behind drownings, as is the failure to wear a life vest when boating.

Accidental falls are a significant cause of death and disability. In 2001, they accounted for more than 15,000 deaths, according to the CDC.

Making It Real

Never drink and drive, and never be the passenger of someone who has been drinking. Resist exceeding 65 mph on the highway, as lower speeds give you a life-saving edge in reaction time. To prevent an accident due to fatigue, if you become sleepy while driving, pull over immediately and take a nap or let someone else drive.

AAA warns drivers to be aware that trucks have blind spots, so when passing them, do so quickly. And don't drive alongside a big rig. As for dealing with aggressive drivers, AAA advises drivers to "swallow your pride" and don't engage with rude, aggressive drivers. Avoid eye contact; otherwise it can turn into a personal duel. Also, while driving beware of distractions, and realize the dangers of even briefly diverting your attention from driving, such as changing a CD or making a cell phone call. Always use your seat belt, and select a car with air bags.

If you bike but don't regularly wear a helmet, develop the habit by purchasing one you find comfortable and good looking. Both factors contribute to higher usage. To prevent an adverse drug reaction, be sure to tell your doctor and pharmacist about any drugs or supplements you're currently taking. Also, check if your doctor's prescription is legible.

To prevent carbon monoxide poisoning, have your fuel-burning appliances checked annually for leaks. Never use in your home fuel-burning appliances intended for the outdoors, as they often emit unsafe levels of carbon monoxide.

And don't leave an engine running in an enclosed space. Be sure to install carbon monoxide alarms at home along with smoke alarms—another proven lifesaver.

Safe water activity tips include not mixing alcohol and swimming. Never swim alone. People of all ages should have someone keeping an eye on them while in the water. And wear a vest when boating, even if you're a strong swimmer.

A number of simple steps can also sharply cut the odds of an accidental fall. These include placing night lights throughout the home, keeping stairways free of clutter, and installing grips in the shower and non-skid strips in the bathtub.

To Learn More

Visit the CDC's National Center for Injury Prevention and Control at www.cdc.gov/ncipc. You can also order information on injury prevention by calling the CDC's public information line at (800) 311-3435. Go the National Safety Council's website at www.nsc.org and click on the "Odds of Dying" icon to view statistics on the leading causes of accidental U.S. deaths.

CHAPTER 50

Don't Dwell on Genes

Genes do matter in the quest for a long life, but plenty of studies show you've still got the upper hand over your genetic endowment.

Between 20 to 30 percent of longevity is attributed to genetic causes, a recent study concluded, based on research on twins raised separately. That leaves at least 70 percent in your control, largely contingent on lifestyle choices. Take a lesson from centenarians about ways to maximize your life span. As a rule, they stay physically active most or all of their lives, remain engaged with friends, and enjoy strong family ties. They're notable "stress-shedders," and rarely smoked during their lives, if at all. One researcher also notes that he's never seen an obese centenarian.

In fact, most people inherit a set of genes that allows them to live well into their eighties, asserts Thomas Perls, MD, MPH, the director of the New England Centenarian Study. And those making an effort to prevent the diseases of aging can add another 10 years, Perls says.

So how does one capture those extra 10 years? Look to the Okinawans in Japan. They have the longest life expectancy worldwide, as well as an unusually large number of centenarians. These people enjoy strong social ties and follow an active lifestyle into old age, while consuming a low-calorie, low-fat diet.

Today's centenarians also had the longevity advantage of growing up in an era when cars were a rarity, television a figment of a few inventors' imaginations, and fast food meant an apple for the road. Reaching a grand old age, it's clear from research, now depends more on rebuffing the temptations of contemporary life than on getting lucky in the genetic lottery.

As Perls states in a 2004 *Time* magazine interview: "Each of us can earn the right to have at least 25 years beyond the age of 60—years of healthy life at good function. The disappointing news is that it requires work and willpower."

What Scientists Know

Studies of long-living populations show convincingly that lifestyle plays a dominant role in setting your life's clock. One study looked at the clean-living Seventh Day Adventists, who eat far less red meat than average Americans, drink and smoke infrequently if at all, and usually take above-average care of their health.

Researchers found up to a 10-year survival advantage among those who followed the best health practices.

Among the most famous diets associated with longevity is that of the Okinawans. These exceptionally long-living people suffer 80 percent fewer heart attacks than Americans. Obesity is rare among them, as are strokes, cancers, osteoporosis, and dementia. The health profile of an elderly Okinawan usually reads like that of a person decades younger: healthy cholesterol levels, low homocysteine, and reasonable blood pressure throughout life, researchers in one study note.

Researchers are confident that the islanders' longevity and freedom from disease are primarily associated with lifestyle, not genetics. They capture those extra 10 years that Perls mentions by consuming fewer calories on average than other Japanese people, and centering their meals on fish, soy-based foods, antioxidant-rich vegetables, fruits, tea, and seaweed. The Okinawans use little salt and rarely smoke. They also engage in regular physical activity, such as farming and dancing, and generally report satisfying relationships with family and other villagers.

Genes undoubtedly play some protective role against many of the diseases of aging, although their pathways haven't been clearly identified. And Perls says genes likely play a role in reaching extreme old age. One study recently reported that brothers of centenarians were 17 times more likely to reach age 100 than the general population, and sisters 8 times more likely.

Making It Real

In his book *Living to 100: Lessons in Living to Your Maximum Potential at Any Age*, Perls outlines strategies for making the most of your genetic endowment. As he writes: "Unfortunately, the vast majority of baby boomers do a terrible job of preparing for old age. High-fat diets, smoking, excessive drinking, and lack of exercise not only reduce people's chances of achieving older age, they markedly increase the likelihood of a longer period of poor health in a shorter life. Yet many of us have the genes to get to old age and perhaps extreme old age. We just have to learn to use them."

Perls emphasizes the approach of "compressing morbidity" into just the final few years of life, if at all. That means if you're going to experience declining health, aim to do so as rapidly and close to the end as possible.

As Perls emphasizes in *Living to 100*, the diligent use of antioxidants can slow age-related diseases like atherosclerosis, cancers and dementia. Maintaining cognitive capacity is closely associated with reaching great old age, so follow guidelines for maintaining mental function, including continually learning through life and remaining engaged in outside affairs. One of the strengths of centenarians was their ability to shed stress—they took life's twists and turns in far better stride than most. If you find yourself coping with too much stress, make sure to exercise regularly to manage it, and explore stress-reduction practices like meditation or Tai Chi. Be sure to monitor markers of health status, such as blood pressure, and cholesterol, homocysteine, triglyceride, and glucose levels.

To Learn More

Read Perls' book, *Living to 100: Lessons in Living to Your Maximum Potential at Any Age.* To use an informative "Living to 100 Life Expectancy Calculator," go the Boston University home page at www.bu.edu and type "Living to 100" in the search box, then select the calculator.

Bibliography

Chapter 1

Blue Shield of California. 2000. *Blue Shield offers a guided imagery program to pre-surgical patients.* www.mylifepath.com.

Bradshaw A, Katzer L, Horwath CC, Gray A, et al. 2004. A randomised trial of three non-dieting programs for overweight women. *Asia Pacific Journal of Clinical Nutrition* 13(Suppl):S43.

Jasnoski ML, Kugler J. 1987. Relaxation, imagery, and neuroimmunomodulation. *Annals of New York Academic Science* 496:722-30.

Kiecolt-Glaser JK, Glaser R, Strain EC, et al. 1986. Modulation of cellular immunity in medical students. *Journal of Behavioral Medicine* 9(1):5-21.

Liggett DR, Hamada S. 1993. Enhancing the visualization of gymnasts. *American Journal of Clinical Hypnosis* 35(3):190-7.

Ornish, Dean, MD. 2004. Interview with the authors. August 5.

Patel C, Marmot MG, Terry DJ, Carruthers M, et al. 1985. Trial of relaxation in reducing coronary risk: four year follow up. *British Medical Journal (Clinical Research Edition)* 290(6475):1103-6.

Patel C, Marmot MG. 1987. Stress management, blood pressure and quality of life. *Journal of Hypertension Supplement* 5(1):S21-8.

Ranganathan VK, Siemionow V, Liu JZ, Sahgal V, Yue GH. 2004. From mental power to muscle power—gaining strength by using the mind. *Neuropsychologia* 42(7):944-56.

Chapter 2

Anson RM, Guo Z, de Cabo R, et al. 2003. Intermittent fasting dissociates beneficial effects of dietary restriction on glucose metabolism and neuronal resistance to injury from calorie intake. *Proceedings of the National Academy of the Sciences of the U.S.A.* 100(10):6216-20.

Mattison JA, Lane MA, Roth GS, Ingram DK. 2003. Calorie restriction in rhesus monkeys. *Experimental Gerontology* 38(1-2):35-46.

Mattson, Mark, PhD. 2003. Interview with the authors. September 10.

McCay, Ed., A.I. Lansing. 1952. *Cowdry's Problems of Aging, Biological and Medical Aspects, C.M.* Baltimore: Williams and Wilkins. 1952, p. 130.

Merry BJ. 2004. Oxidative stress and mitochondrial function with aging—the effects of calorie restriction. *Aging Cell* 3(1):7-12.

Scrofano MM, Shang F, Nowell TR Jr, et al. 1998. Calorie restriction, stress and the ubiquitin-dependent pathway in mouse livers. *Mechanisms of Aging and Development* 105(3):273-90.

Swan PB. 1997. To live longer, eat less! (McCay, 1934-1939). *Journal of Nutrition* 127(5 Suppl):1039S-1041S.

Yamori Y, Miura A, Taira K. 2001. Implications from and for food cultures for cardiovascular diseases: Japanese food, particularly Okinawan diets. *Asia Pacific Journal of Clinical Nutrition* 10(2):144-5.

Chapter 3

Anson RM, Guo Z, Mattson MP, et al. 2003. Intermittent fasting dissociates beneficial effects of dietary restriction on glucose metabolism and neuronal resistance to injury from calorie intake. *Proceedings of the National Academy of the Sciences of the U.S.A.* 100(10):6216-20.

Mattson, Mark, PhD. 2003. Interview with the authors. September 10.

Wan R, Camandola S, Mattson MP. 2003. Intermittent fasting and dietary supplementation with 2-deoxy-D-glucose improve functional and metabolic cardiovascular risk factors in rats. *The FASEB Journal* 17(9):1133-4.

Chapter 4

Colcombe SJ, Kramer AF, McAuley E, Erickson KI, Scalf P. J. 2004. Neurocognitive aging and cardiovascular fitness: recent findings and future directions. *Molecular Neuroscience* 24(1):9-14.

Feskanich D, Willett W, Colditz G. 2002.Walking and leisure-time activity and risk of hip fracture in postmenopausal women. *Journal of the American Medical Association* 288(18):2300-6.

Lee IM, Paffenbarger RS Jr. 1998. Physical activity and stroke incidence: the Harvard Alumni Health Study. *Stroke* 29(10):2049-54.

Lee IM, Rexrode KM, Cook NR, Manson JE, Buring JE. 2001 Physical activity and coronary heart disease in women: is "no pain, no gain" passe? *Journal of the American Medical Association* 285(11):1447-54.

Manson JE, Hu FB, Rich-Edwards JW, Colditz GA, et al. 1999. A prospective study of walking as compared with vigorous exercise in the prevention of coronary heart disease in women. *New England Journal of Medicine* 341(9):650-8.

Chapter 5

Brickey, Michael, PhD, 2004. Interview with the authors. August 18.

Hausdorff J., Levy B. & Wei J. 1999. The power of ageism on physical function of older persons: Reversibility of age-related gait changes. *Journal of the American Geriatric Society* 47:1346-1349.

Levy, Becca, PhD. 2004. Interview with the authors. July 28.

Levy B. 1996. Improving memory in old age by implicit self-stereotyping. *Journal of Personality and Social Psychology* 71:1092-1107.

Levy B. & Langer E. 1994. Aging free from negative stereotypes: Successful memory among the American Deaf and in China. *Journal of Personality and Social Psychology* 66:935-943.

Levy BR, Hausdorff JM, Hencke R, Wei JY. 2000. Reducing cardiovascular stress with positive self-stereotypes of aging. *Journal of Gerontology. Series B Psychological Science and Social Science* 55(4):P205-13.

Levy BR, Slade MD, Kunkel SR, Kasl SV. 2002. Longevity increased by positive self-perceptions of aging. *Journal of Personal Social Psychology* 83(2):261-70.

Chapter 6

Ames B. 2001. DNA damage from micronutrient deficiencies is likely to be a major cause of cancer. *Mutation Research* (475)7-20.

Ballmer PE, Stahelin HB. 1994. Beta carotene, vitamin E, and lung cancer. *New England Journal of Medicine* 330(15):1029-35.

Blumberg, Jeffrey, PhD. 2004. Interview with the authors. May 10.

Dowd P, Zheng ZB. 1995. On the mechanism of the anticlotting action of vitamin E quinone. *Proceedings of the National Academy of the Sciences of the U.S.A.* 92(18):8171-5.

Fletcher RH, Fairfield KM. 2002. Vitamins for chronic disease prevention in adults: clinical applications. *Journal of the American Medical Association* 287(23):3127-9.

Horwitt, Max K. 1974. Status of human requirements for vitamin E. *American Journal of Clinical Nutrition* 27:1182-93.

Oski, F. A. and Barness, L. A. 1967. Vitamin E deficiency: A previously unrecognized cause of hemolytic anemia in the premature infant. *Journal of Pediatrics* 70:211-20.

Pryor WA. 2000. Vitamin E and heart disease: basic science to clinical intervention trials. *Free Radical Biological Medicine* 28(1):141-64.

Chapter 7

Bredie SJ, Wollersheim H, Verheugt FW, Thien T. 2003. Low-dose aspirin for primary prevention of cardiovascular disease. *Seminars of Vascular Medicine* 3(2):177-84.

Corley DA, Kerlikowske K, Verma R, Buffler P. 2003. Protective association of aspirin/NSAIDSs and esophageal cancer: a systematic review and meta-analysis. *Gastroenterology* 124(1):47-56.

Cornelius C, Fastbom J, Winblad B, Viitanen M. 2004. Aspirin, NSAIDS risk of dementia, and influence of the apolipoprotein E epsilon 4 allele in an elderly population.. *Neuroepidemiology* 23(3):135-43.

Drake JG, Becker JL. 2002. Aspirin-induced inhibition of ovarian tumor cell growth. *American Journal of Obstetric Gynecology* 100(4):677-82.

Harris RE, Beebe-Donk J, Namboodiri KK, et al. 2001. Inverse association of non-steroidal anti-inflammatory drugs and malignant melanoma among women. *Oncology Reports* 8(3):655-7.

Hayden M, Pignone M, Phillips C, Mulrow C. 2002. Aspirin for the primary prevention of cardiovascular events: a summary of the evidence for the U.S. Preventive Services Task Force. *Annals of Internal Medicine* 136(2):I55.

Kasum CM, Blair CK, Folsom AR, Ross JA. 2003. Non-steroidal anti-inflammatory drug use and risk of adult leukemia. *Cancer Epidemiology, Biomarkers and Prevention* 12(6):534-7.

Khuder SA, Mutgi AB. 2001. Breast cancer and NSAIDS use: a meta-analysis. *British Journal of Cancer* 84(9):1188-92.

Kim ES, Hong WK, Khuri FR. 2002. Chemoprevention of aerodigestive tract cancers. *Annual Review of Medicine* 53:223-43.

Kirschenbaum A, Liu X, Yao S, Levine AC. 2001. The role of cyclooxygenase-2 in prostate cancer. *Urology* 58(2 Suppl 1):127-31.

Lieberman R. 2002. Chemoprevention of prostate cancer: current status and future directions. *Cancer Metastasis Review* 21:297–309.

Nilsson SE, Johansson B, Takkinen S, et al. 2003. Does aspirin protect against Alzheimer's dementia? A study in a Swedish population-based sample aged > or = 80 years. *European Journal of Clinical Pharmacology* 59(4):313-9.

Rollet J. 2004. The miracle in the cabinet. A look at the future of aspirin. *Advance for Nurse Practitioners* 12(3):91-3.

Terry MB, Gammon MD, Zhang FF, et al. 2004. Association of frequency and duration of aspirin use and hormone receptor status with breast cancer risk. *Journal of the American Medical Association* 291(20):2488-9.

Thun, Michael, MD. 2004. Interview with the authors. July 28.

2003. Aspirin for everything? *Consumer Reports* 68(7):51.

Chapter 8

Stafford RS, Drieling RL, Hersh AL. 2004. National trends in osteoporosis visits and osteoporosis treatment: 1988 – 2003. *Archives of Internal Medicine* July 26.

Calbet JA, Moysi JS, Dorado C, Rodriguez LP. 1998. Bone mineral content and density in professional tennis players. *Calcified Tissue International* 62(6):491-6.

Calvo MS, Whiting SJ. 2003. Prevalence of vitamin D insufficiency in Canada and the United States: importance to health status and efficacy of current food fortification and dietary supplement use. *Nutrition Reviews* 61(3):107-13.

Feskanich D, Weber P, Willett WC, Rockett H, Booth SL, Colditz GA. 1999. Vitamin K intake and hip fractures in women: a prospective study. *American Journal of Clinical Nutrition* 69(1):74-9.

Feskanich D, Willett WC, Stampfer MJ, Colditz GA. 1996. Protein consumption and bone fractures in women. *American Journal of Epidemiology* 143(5):472-9.

Feskanich, Diane, ScD. 2004. Interview with the authors. August 24.

Holick MF. 2003. Vitamin D: A millenium perspective. *Journal of Cellular Biochemistry* 88(2):296-307.

Kostuik JP, Jandebeur SM, Margolis S. 2004. Back Pain and Osteoporosis. 2004. *Johns Hopkins White Papers*.

Messina M, Gardner C, Barnes S. 2002. Gaining insight into the health effects of soy but a long way still to go. *Journal of Nutrition* 132(3):547S-551S.

Michaelsson K, Lithell H, Vessby B, Melhus H. 2003. Serum retinol levels and the risk of fracture. *New England Journal of Medicine* 23348(4):287-94.

National Institutes of Health Fact Sheets: "Nutrition and the Skeleton," "What is Bone?" "Phytoestrogens and Bone Health," and "Osteoporosis and Men." www.osteo.org/osteolinks.asp.

National Osteoporosis Foundation. 2004. Prevention: Exercise for Healthy Bones. www.nof.org/prevention/exercise.htm.
"National Osteoporosis Foundation Releases Survey Showing Few Women Believe They Are at Risk for Osteoporosis, Despite Staggering Prevalence Numbers." Press release, www.nof.org/news/pressreleases/2004_health_issues_survey.htm (accessed April 6, 2004).

Promislow JH, Goodman-Gruen D, Slymen DJ, Barrett-Connor E. 2002. Protein consumption and bone mineral density in the elderly: the Rancho Bernardo Study. *American Journal of Epidemiology* 155(7):636-44.

van Meurs JB, Dhonukshe-Rutten RA, Pluijm SM, et al. 2004. Homocysteine levels and the risk of osteoporotic fractures. *New England Journal of Medicine* May 13.

Chapter 9

Egolf B, Lasker J, Wolf S, Potvin L. 1992. The Roseto effect: a 50-year comparison of mortality rates. *American Journal of Public Health* 82(8):1089-92.

Keys A. 1966. Arteriosclerotic heart disease in Roseto, Pennsylvania. *Journal of the American Medical Association* 195(2):93-5.

Kravdal O. 2001. The impact of marital status on cancer survival. *Social Science and Medicine* 52(3):357-68.

Seeman TE. 1996. Social ties and health: the benefits of social integration. *Annals of Epidemiology* 6(5):442-51.

Shaffer, Carolyn. 2004. Interview with the authors. August 28.

Williams RB, Barefoot JC, Califf RM, Haney TL, et al. 1992. Prognostic importance of social and economic resources among medically treated patients with angiographically documented coronary artery disease. *Journal of the American Medical Association* 267(4):520-4.

Wingard DL, Berkman LF, Brand RJ. 1982. A multivariate analysis of health-related practices: a nine-year mortality follow-up of the Alameda County Study. *American Journal of Epidemiology* 116(5):765-75.

Chapter 10

Brown SL, Nesse RM, Vinokur AD, Smith DM. 2003. Providing social support may be more beneficial than receiving it: results from a prospective study of mortality. *Psychological Science* 14(4):320-7.

Brown, Stephanie, PhD. 2003. Interview with the authors. June 30.

Musick MA, Herzog AR, House JS. 1999. Volunteering and mortality among older adults: findings from a national sample. *Journal of Gerontology. Series B Psychological Science and Social Science* 54(3):S173-80.

Shmotkin D, Blumstein T, Modan B. 2003. Beyond keeping active: concomitants of being a volunteer in old-old age. *Psychology and Aging* 18(3):602-7.

Chapter 11

Chung FL, Schwartz J, Herzog CR, Yang YM. 2003. Tea and cancer prevention: studies in animals and humans. *Journal of Nutrition* 133(10):3268S-3274S.

Huxley RR, Neil HA. 2003. The relation between dietary flavonol intake and coronary heart disease mortality: a meta-analysis of prospective cohort studies. *European Journal of Clinical Nutrition* 57(8):904-8.

Linden KG, Carpenter PM, McLaren CE. 2003. Chemoprevention of nonmelanoma skin cancer: experience with a polyphenol from green tea. *Recent Results in Cancer Research* 163:165-71.

Nance CL, Shearer WT. 2003. Is green tea good for HIV-1 infection?. *Journal of Allergy and Clinical Immunology* 112(5):951-7.

Sartippour MR, Shao ZM, Heber D, Beatty P, et al. 2002. Green tea inhibits vascular endothelial growth factor (VEGF) induction in human breast cancer cells. *Journal of Nutrition* 132(8):2307-11.

Sueoka N, Suganuma M, Sueoka E, Okabe S. 2001. A new function of green tea: prevention of lifestyle-related diseases. *Annals of New York Academic Science* 928:274-80.

Weisburger JH. 1999. Second international scientific symposium on tea and human health: An introduction. *Proceedings of the Society for Experimental Biology and Medicine* 220(4):193-4.

Weisburger JH. 2002. Lifestyle, health and disease prevention: the underlying mechanisms. *European Journal of Cancer Prevention* 11 Supplement 2:S1-7.

Weisburger, John H., MD, PhD. Interview with the authors. April 8.

Wu AH, Yu MC, Tseng CC, Hankin J, Pike MC. 2003. Green tea and risk of breast cancer in Asian Americans. *International Journal of Cancer* 106(4):574-9.

2004. Component in green tea helps kill leukemia cells. *Mayo Clinic Women's Healthsource* 8(9):3.

Chapter 12

Christenfeld N, Gerin W, Linden W., et al. 1997. Social support effects on cardiovascular reactivity: is a stranger as effective as a friend? *Psychosomatic Medicine* 59(4):388-98.

Davis H, Levine S. 1982. Predictability, control, and the pituitary-adrenal response in rats. *Journal of Comparative and Physiological Psychology* 96(3):393-404.

Herrmann TF, Hurwitz HM, Levine S. 1984. Behavioral control, aversive stimulus frequency, and pituitary-adrenal response. *Behavioral Neuroscience* 98(6):1094-9.

Levine S. 2000. Influence of psychological variables on the activity of the hypothalamic-pituitary-adrenal axis. *European Journal of Pharmacology* 405(1-3):149-60.

Perls T., Hutter Silver M. 1999. *Living to 100: Lessons in Living to Your Maximum Potential at Any Age.* New York: Basic Books, 1999. "they're what researchers term 'stress shedders.'" p. 167.

Rubinstein JS, Meyer DE, Evans JE. 2001. Executive control of cognitive processes in task switching. *Journal of Experimental Psychology. Human Perception and Performance* 27(4):763-97.

Sapolsky, Robert M., PhD. 2004. Interview with the authors. Sept. 24.

Sapolsky, Robert M. 1998. *Why Zebras Don't Get Ulcers: An Updated Guide to Stress, Stress-Related Diseases, and Coping.* New York: W.H. Freeman, 1998.

Schuler JL, O'Brien WH. 1997. Cardiovascular recovery from stress and hypertension risk factors: a meta-analytic review. *Psychophysiology* 34(6):649-59.

Walton KG, Schneider RH, Nidich S. 2004. Review of controlled research on the transcendental meditation program and cardiovascular disease. Risk factors, morbidity, and mortality. *Cardiology in Review* 12(5):262-6.

Chapter 13

Hawley JA. 2004. Exercise as a therapeutic intervention for the prevention and treatment of insulin resistance. *Diabetes/Metabolism Research and Review* 20(5):383-93.

Jakicic JM. 2002. The role of physical activity in prevention and treatment of body weight gain in adults. *Journal of Nutrition* 132(12):3826S-3829S.

La Lanne, Jack. 2004. www.jacklalanne.com.

Lee IM, Paffenbarger RS Jr. 1998. Physical activity and stroke incidence: the Harvard Alumni Health Study. *Stroke* 29(10):2049-54.

Manson JE, Greenland P, LaCroix AZ, et al. 2002. Walking compared with vigorous exercise for the prevention of cardiovascular events in women. *New England Journal of Medicine* 347(10):716-25.

McTiernan A. 2003. Physical activity, exercise, and cancer: prevention to treatment—symposium overview. *Medicine and Science in Sports and Exercise* 35(11):1821-2.

Meyer T, Broocks A. 2000. Therapeutic impact of exercise on psychiatric diseases: guidelines for exercise testing and prescription. *Sports Medicine* 30(4):269-79.

Myers J, Prakash M, Froelicher V, et al. 2002. Exercise capacity and mortality among men referred for exercise testing. *New England Journal of Medicine* 346(11):793-801.

Potteiger, Jeffrey A., PhD. 2004. Interview with the authors. October 14.

Rollo, I. 2004. Understanding the role of exercise in health promotion. *Nursing Times* 100(37):36-8.

Stein RA, Chesler R, Safi AM. 2001 Exercise update 2001. *Heart Disease* 3(5):306-12.

Tworoger SS, Yasui Y, Vitiello MV, Schwartz RS, et al. 2003. Effects of a yearlong moderate-intensity exercise and a stretching intervention on sleep quality in postmenopausal women. *Sleep* 26(7):830-6.

Vainionpaa A, Korpelainen R, Leppaluoto J, Jamsa T. 2004. Effects of high-impact exercise on bone mineral density: a randomized controlled trial in premenopausal women. *Osteoporosis International* June 17.

Chapter 14

Buckwalter JA. 1997. Maintaining and restoring mobility in middle and old age: the importance of soft tissues. *Instructional course lectures* 46:459-469. Rosemont, IL, American Academy of Orthopaedic Surgeons, 1997.

Feigenbaum MS, Pollock ML. 1999. Prescription of resistance training for health and disease. *Medicine and Science in Sports and Exercise* 31(1):38-45.

Fiatarone, MA, Marks EC, Ryan ND, et al. 1990. High-intensity training in nonagenarians: effects of skeletal muscle. *Journal of the American Medical Association* 23(22):3029-3034.

Holten MK, Zacho M, Gaster M, et al. 2004. Strength training increases insulin-mediated glucose uptake, GLUT4 content, and insulin signaling in skeletal muscle in patients with type 2 diabetes. *Diabetes* 53(2):294-305.

Kelley GA, Kelley KS. 2000. Progressive resistance exercise and resting blood pressure: A meta-analysis of randomized controlled trials. *Hypertension* 35(3):838-43.

Nelson ME, Fiatarone MA, Morganti CM, Trice I, Greenberg RA, Evans WJ. 1994. Effects of high-intensity strength training on multiple risk factors for osteoporotic fractures. A randomized controlled trial. *Journal of the American Medical Association* 272(24):1909-14.

Potteiger, Jeffrey A. PhD. 2004. Interview with the authors. October 14.

Rosenberg, Irwin, MD. 2004. Interview with the authors. August 11.

Seynnes O, Fiatarone Singh MA, Hue O, Pras P, et al. 2004. Physiological and functional responses to low-moderate versus high-intensity progressive resistance training in frail elders. *Journal of Gerontology. Series A, Biological Sciences and Medical Sciences* 59(5):503-9.

Singh NA, Clements KM, Fiatarone MA. 1997. A randomized controlled trial of the effect of exercise on sleep. *Sleep* 20(2):95-101.

Singh NA, Clements KM, Fiatarone MA. 1997. A randomized controlled trial of progressive resistance training in depressed elders. *Journal of Gerontology. Series A, Biological Sciences and Medical Sciences* 52(1):M27-35.

Tseng BS, Marsh DR, Hamilton MT, Booth FW. 1995. Strength and aerobic training attenuate muscle wasting and improve resistance to the development of disability with aging. *Journal of Gerontology. Series A, Biological Sciences and Medical Sciences* 50 Spec No:113-9.

Winett RA, Carpinelli RN. 2001. Potential health-related benefits of resistance training. *Preventitive Medicine* 33(5):503-13.

Chapter 15

Carlsson CM, Pharo LM, Aeschlimann SE, et al. 2004. Effects of multivitamins and low-dose folic acid supplements on flow-mediated vasodilation and plasma homocysteine levels in older adults. *American Heart Journal* 148(3):E11.

Homocysteine Studies Collaboration. 2002. Homocysteine and risk of ischemic heart disease and stroke: a meta-analysis. *Journal of the American Medical Association* 288(16):2015-22.

Hu, FB, et al. 2000. Prospective study of major dietary patterns of risk of coronary heart disease in men. *American Journal of Clinical Nutrition* 72:912-21.

Katz DL. 2004. Lifestyle and dietary modification for prevention of heart failure. *The Medical Clinics of North America* 88(5):1295-320.

Miller M, Cosgrove B, Havas S. 2002. Update on the role of triglycerides as a risk factor for coronary heart disease. *Current Atherosclerosis Reports* 4(6):414-8.

Mori TA, Beilin LJ. 2004. Omega-3 Fatty acids and inflammation. *Current Atherosclerosis Reports* 6(6):461-7.

Renaud S, de Lorgeril M. 1992. Wine, alcohol, platelets, and the French paradox for coronary heart disease. *Lancet* 339(8808):1523-6.

Spratt KA. 2004. Reducing the risk of coronary heart disease via lipid reduction. *Journal of the American Osteopathic Association* 104(9 Suppl 7):S9-13.

Vrentzos G, Papadakis JA, Malliaraki N, et al. 2004. Association of serum total homocysteine with the extent of ischemic heart disease in a Mediterranean cohort. *Angiology* 55(5):517-24.

Chapter 16

Andreassen AK, Hartmann A, Offstad J, et al. 1997. Hypertension prophylaxis with omega-3 fatty acids in heart transplant recipients. *Journal of the American College of Cardiology* 29(6):1324-31.

DASH-Sodium Collaborative Research Group. Sacks FM, Svetkey LP, Vollmer WM, et al. 2001. Effects on blood pressure of reduced dietary sodium and the Dietary Approaches to Stop Hypertension (DASH) diet. *New England Journal of Medicine* 344(1):3-10.

Kearney PM, Whelton M, Reynolds K, et al. 2004. Worldwide prevalence of hypertension: a systematic review. *Journal of Hypertension* 22(1):11-9.

Krousel-Wood MA, Muntner P, He J, Whelton PK. 2004. Primary prevention of essential hypertension. *The Medical Clinics of North America* 88(1):223-38.

Landsbergis PA, Schnall PL, Belkic KL, et al. 2001. Work stressors and cardiovascular disease. *Work* 17(3):191-208.

Law M. 2000. Salt, blood pressure, and cardiovascular diseases. *Journal of Cardiovascular Risk* 7(1):5-8.

Li YC, Qiao G, Uskokovic M, Xiang W, et al. 2004. Vitamin D: a negative endocrine regulator of the renin-angiotensin system and blood pressure. *Journal of Steroid Biochemistry and Molecular Biology* 89-90(1-5):387-92.

Linden W, Lenz JW, Con AH. 2001. Individualized stress management for primary hypertension: a randomized trial. *Archives of Internal Medicine* 161(8):1071-80.

Stevens VJ, Obarzanek E, Cook NR, et al. 2001. Long-term weight loss and changes in blood pressure: results of the Trials of Hypertension Prevention, phase II. *Annals of Internal Medicine* 134(1):1-11.

Sudsuang R, Chentanez V, Veluvan K. 1991. Effect of Buddhist meditation on serum cortisol and total protein levels, blood pressure, pulse rate, lung volume, and reaction time. *Physiology and Behavior* 50(3):543-8.

Tsai JC, Yang HY, Wang WH, et al. 2004. The beneficial effect of regular endurance exercise training on blood pressure and quality of life in patients with hypertension. *Clinical and Experimental Hypertension* 26(3):255-65.

Whelton PK, He J, Cutler JA, et al. 1997. Effects of oral potassium on blood pressure. Meta-analysis of randomized controlled clinical trials. *Journal of the American Medical Association* 277(20):1624-1632.

Whelton, Paul K., MD, MSc. 2004. Interview with the authors. Nov. 16.

Chapter 17

Castaneda C, Layne JE, Munoz-Orians L, et al. 2002. A randomized controlled trial of resistance exercise training to improve glycemic control in older adults with type 2 diabetes. *Diabetes Care* 25(12):2335-41.

Knowler WC, Barrett-Connor E, Fowler SE, et al. 2002. Reduction in the incidence of type 2 diabetes with lifestyle intervention or metformin. *New England Journal of Medicine* 346(6):393-403.

Klein S, Sheard NF, Pi-Sunyer, et al. 2004.Weight management through lifestyle modification for the prevention and management of type 2 diabetes: rationale and strategies. A statement of the American Diabetes Association, the North American Association for the Study of Obesity, and the American Society for Clinical Nutrition. *American Journal of Clinical Nutrition* 80(2):257-63X.

Salmeron J, Hu FB, Manson JE, et al. 2001. Dietary fat intake and risk of type 2 diabetes in women. *American Journal of Clinical Nutrition.* 73(6):1019-26.

Schulze MB, Hu FB. 2004. Primary Prevention of Diabetes: What Can Be Done and How Much Can Be Prevented? *Annual Review of Public Health* Oct 26.

Spiegel K, Leproult R, Van Cauter E. 1999. Impact of sleep debt on metabolic and endocrine function. Lancet 354(9188):1435-9.

Thorsdottir I, Hill J, Ramel A. 2004. Omega-3 fatty acid supply from milk associates with lower type 2 diabetes in men and coronary heart disease in women. *Preventitive Medicine* 39(3):630-4.

Tibbetts, Cathy, CDE. 2004. Interview with the authors. November 23.

Van de Wiel A. 2004. Diabetes mellitus and alcohol. *Diabetes/Metabolism Research and Review* (4):263-7.

Chapter 18

Baron JA, Cole BF, Sandler RS, et al. 2003. A randomized trial of aspirin to prevent colorectal adenomas. *New England Journal of Medicine* 348(10):891-9.

Calcium Polyp Prevention Study Group. Baron JA, Beach M, Mandel JS, et al. 1999. Calcium supplements for the prevention of colorectal adenomas. *New England Journal of Medicine* 340(2):101-7.

Cho E, Smith-Warner SA, Spiegelman D, et al. 2004. Dairy foods, calcium, and colorectal cancer: a pooled analysis of 10 cohort studies. *Journal of the National Cancer Institute* 96(13):1015-22.

Cram P, Fendrick AM, Inadomi J, et al. 2003. The impact of a celebrity promotional campaign on the use of colon cancer screening: the Katie Couric effect. *Archives of Internal Medicine* 163(13):1601-5.

Cross AJ, Sinha R. 2004. Meat-related mutagens/carcinogens in the etiology of colorectal cancer. *Environmental and Molecular Mutagenesis* 44(1):44-55.

Fuchs CS, Giovannucci EL, Colditz GA, et al. 1999. Dietary fiber and the risk of colorectal cancer and adenoma in women. *New England Journal of Medicine* 340(3):169-76.

Glade, MJ. 1999. *Food, Nutrition and the Prevention of Cancer: a global perspective,* 1997. Nutrition 15(6):523-6.

Meyers, Samuel, MD. 2004. Interview with the authors. November 24.

Peters U, Sinha R, Chatterjee N, et al. 2003. Dietary fibre and colorectal adenoma in a colorectal cancer early detection programme. *Lancet* 361(9368):1491-5.

Phoenix Colon Cancer Prevention Physicians' Network. Alberts DS, Martinez ME, Roe DJ, et al. 2000. Lack of effect of a high-fiber cereal supplement on the recurrence of colorectal adenomas. *New England Journal of Medicine* 342(16):1156-62.

Pickhardt PJ, Choi JR, Hwang I, et al. 2003. Computed tomographic virtual colonoscopy to screen for colorectal neoplasia in asymptomatic adults. *New England Journal of Medicine* 349(23):2191-200.

Terry P, Jain M, Miller AB, et al. 2002. Dietary intake of folic acid and colorectal cancer risk in a cohort of women. *International Journal of Cancer* 97(6):864-7.

Jacobs ET, Jiang R, Alberts DS, et al. 2004. Selenium and colorectal adenoma: results of a pooled analysis. *Journal of the National Cancer Institute* 96(22):1669-75.

Feskanich D, Ma J, Fuchs CS, et al. 2004. Plasma vitamin D metabolites and risk of colorectal cancer in women. *Cancer Epidemiology, Biomarkers and Prevention* 13(9):1502-8.

Chapter 19

Carroll, Peter, MD. 2004. Interview with the authors. October 8.

Giovannucci E, Ascherio A, Rimm EB, et al. 1995. Intake of carotenoids and retinol in relation to risk of prostate cancer. *Journal of the National Cancer Institute* 87(23):1767-76.

Giovannucci E. 2002. A review of epidemiologic studies of tomatoes, lycopene, and prostate cancer. *Experimental Biology and Medicine (Maywood)* 227(10):852-9.

Kucuk O, Sarkar FH, Sakr W, et al. 2001. Phase II randomized clinical trial of lycopene supplementation before radical prostatectomy. *Cancer Epidemiology, Biomarkers and Prevention* 10(8):861-8.

Leitzmann MF, Platz EA, Stampfer MJ, et al. 2004. Ejaculation frequency and subsequent risk of prostate cancer. *Journal of the American Medical Association* 291(13):1578-86.

Nutritional Prevention of Cancer Study Group. Clark LC, Combs GF Jr, Turnbull BW, et al. 1996. Effects of selenium supplementation for cancer prevention in patients with carcinoma of the skin. A randomized controlled trial. *Journal of the American Medical Association* 276(24):1957-63.

Stewart LV, Weigel NL. 2004. Vitamin D and prostate cancer. *Experimental Biology and Medicine (Maywood)* 229(4):277-84.

Whittemore AS, Kolonel LN, Wu AH, et al. 1995. Prostate cancer in relation to diet, physical activity, and body size in blacks, whites, and Asians in the United States and Canada. *Journal of the National Cancer Institute* 87(9):652-61.

Zhou JR, Yu L, Zhong Y, Blackburn GL. 2003. Soy phytochemicals and tea bioactive components synergistically inhibit androgen-sensitive human prostate tumors in mice. *Journal of Nutrition* 133(2):516-21.

Chapter 20

Brown, Coralie J.P. 2004. Interview with the authors. October 21.

Cho S, Dietrich M, Brown CJ, Clark CA, et al. 2003. The effect of breakfast type on total daily energy intake and body mass index: results from the Third National Health and Nutrition Examination Survey (NHANES III). *Journal of the American College of Nutrition* 22(4):296-302.

Johnson MA, Brown MA, Poon LW, et al. 1992. Nutritional patterns of centenarians. *International Journal of Aging and Human Development* 34(1):57-76.

Karelia, Finland. Kleemola P, Puska P, Vartiainen E, et al. 1999. The effect of breakfast cereal on diet and serum cholesterol: a randomized trial *North European Journal of Clinical Nutrition* 53(9):716-21.

Kleinman RE, Hall S, Green H, et al. 2002. Diet, breakfast, and academic performance in children. *Annals of Nutrition and Metabolism* 46 (Suppl) 1:24-30.

Ma Y, Bertone ER, Stanek EJ 3rd, et al. 2003. Association between eating patterns and obesity in a free-living US adult population. *American Journal of Epidemiology* 158(1):85-92.

Miller HE, Rigelhof F, Marquart L, et al. 2000. Antioxidant content of whole grain breakfast cereals, fruits and vegetables. *Journal of the American College of Nutrition* 19(3 Suppl):312S-319S.

Morgan KJ, Zabik ME, Stampley GL. 1986. The role of breakfast in diet adequacy of the U.S. adult population. *Journal of the American College of Nutrition* 5(6):551-63.

Saltzman E, Das SK, Lichtenstein AH, et al. 2001. An oat-containing hypocaloric diet reduces systolic blood pressure and improves lipid profile beyond effects of weight loss in men and women. *Journal of Nutrition* 131(5):1465-70.

Smith AP. 2002. Stress, breakfast cereal consumption and cortisol. *Nutrition and Neuroscience* 5(2):141-4.

Smith AP. Breakfast and mental health. 1998. *International Journal of Food Sciences and Nutrition* 49(5):397-402.

Tucker KL, Olson B, Bakun P, Dallal GE, et al. 2004. Breakfast cereal fortified with folic acid, vitamin B-6, and vitamin B-12 increases vitamin concentrations and reduces homocysteine concentrations: a randomized trial. *American Journal of Clinical Nutrition* 79(5):805-11.

Wesnes KA, Pincock C, Richardson D, et al. 2003. Breakfast reduces declines in attention and memory over the morning in schoolchildren. *Appetite* 41(3):329-31.

Chapter 21

Demark-Wahnefried W, Rock CL. 2003. Nutrition-related issues for the breast cancer survivor. *Seminars on Oncology* 30(6):789-98.

Gago-Dominguez M, Yuan JM, Sun CL, et al. 2003. Opposing effects of dietary n-3 and n-6 fatty acids on mammary carcinogenesis: The Singapore Chinese Health Study. *British Journal of Cancer* 89(9):1686-92.

Holmes MD, Willett WC. 2004. Does diet affect breast cancer risk? *Breast Cancer Research* 6(4):170-8. Epub June 17.

Kumar N, Allen K, Riccardi D, Kazi A, et al. 2004. Isoflavones in breast cancer chemoprevention: where do we go from here? *Frontiers in Bioscience* 9:2927-34.

Love, Susan M., MD. 2004. Interview with the authors. September 7.

McGregor BA, Bowen DJ, Ankerst DP. 2004. Optimism, perceived risk of breast cancer, and cancer worry among a community-based sample of women. *Health Psychology* 23(4):339-44.

McTiernan A, Kooperberg C, White E, et al. 2003. Recreational physical activity and the risk of breast cancer in postmenopausal women: the Women's Health Initiative Cohort Study. *Journal of the American Medical Association* 290(10):1331-6.

O'Kelly J, Koeffler HP. 2003. Vitamin D analogs and breast cancer. *Recent Results in Cancer Research* 164:333-48.

Rock CL, Demark-Wahnefried W. 2002. Nutrition and survival after the diagnosis of breast cancer: a review of the evidence. *Journal of Clinical Oncology* 20(15):3302-16.

Terry MB, Gammon MD, Zhang FF, et al. 2004. Association of frequency and duration of aspirin use and hormone receptor status with breast cancer risk. *Journal of the American Medical Association* 291(20):2433-40.

Wu AH, Tseng CC, Van Den Berg D, et al. 2003. Tea intake, COMT genotype, and breast cancer in Asian-American women. *Cancer Research* 63(21):7526-9.

Zhang SM, Willett WC, Selhub J, et al. 2003. Plasma folate, vitamin B6, vitamin B12, homocysteine, and risk of breast cancer. *Journal of the National Cancer Institute* 95(5):373-80.

Zhang SM. 2004. Role of vitamins in the risk, prevention, and treatment of breast cancer. *Current Opinions in Obstetrics and Gynecology*

16(1):19-25.

Chapter 22

Badve S. 2004. Ductal lavage and its histopathologic basis: a cautionary tale. *Diagnostic Cytopathology* 30(3):166-71.

Benson SR, Blue J, Judd K, Harman JE. 2004. Ultrasound is now better than mammography for the detection of invasive breast cancer. *American Journal of Surgery* 188(4):381-5.

Kriege M, Brekelmans CT, Boetes C, et al. 2004. Efficacy of MRI and mammography for breast-cancer screening in women with a familial or genetic predisposition. *New England Journal of Medicine* 351(5):497-500.

Love, Susan M., MD. 2004. Interview with the authors. September 7.

Penhoet EE. 2004. Saving Women's Lives: Strategies for Improving Breast Cancer Detection and Diagnosis. *The Institute of Medicine and National Research Council of the National Academies.*

Smith AP, Hall PA, Marcello DM. 2004. Emerging technologies in breast cancer detection. *Radiology Management* 26(4):16-24.

Chapter 23

Baum M. 2004. Does the act of surgery provoke activation of "latent" metastases in early breast cancer? *Breast Cancer Research* 6(4):160-1. Epub 2004 June 09.

Baumgartner RN. 2000. Body composition in healthy aging. *Annals of New York Academic Science* 904:437-48.

Evans WJ. 1996. Reversing sarcopenia: how weight training can build strength and vitality. *Geriatrics* 51(5):46-7, 51-3.

Evans WJ. What is sarcopenia? 1995. *Journal of Gerontology. Series A, Biological Sciences and Medical Sciences* 50 Spec No:5-8.

Fiatarone MA, O'Neill EF, Ryan ND, et al. 1994. Exercise training and nutritional supplementation for physical frailty in very elderly people. *New England Journal of Medicine* 330(25):1769-75.

Frontera WR, Meredith CN, O'Reilly KP, et al. 1988. Strength conditioning in older men: skeletal muscle hypertrophy and improved function. *Journal of Applied Physiology* 64(3):1038-44.

Greenspan SL, Myers ER, Maitland LA, et al. 1994. Fall severity and bone mineral density as risk factors for hip fracture in ambulatory elderly. *Journal of the American Medical Association* 271(2):128-33.

Harris T, Cook DG, Victor C, et al. 2003. Predictors of depressive symptoms in older people—a survey of two general practice populations. *Age and Ageing* 32(5):510-8.

Hurley BF. 1995. Age, gender, and muscular strength. *Journal of Gerontology. Series A, Biological Sciences and Medical Sciences* 50 Spec

No:41-4.

Janssen I, Shepard DS, Katzmarzyk PT, et al. 2004. The healthcare costs of sarcopenia in the United States *Journal of the American Geriatric Society* 52(1):80-5.

Miller AB, To T, Baines CJ, Wall C. 2002. The Canadian National Breast Screening Study-1: breast cancer mortality after 11 to 16 years of follow-up. A randomized screening trial of mammography in women age 40 to 49 years. *Annals of Internal Medicine* 137(5 Part 1):305-12.

Rosenberg, Irwin, MD. 2004. Interview with the authors. August 11.

Tabar L, Yen MF, Vitak B, et al. 2003. Mammography service screening and mortality in breast cancer patients: 20-year follow-up before and after introduction of screening. *Lancet* 361(9367):1405-10.

Chapter 24

Bischoff-Ferrari HA, Dawson-Hughes B, Willett WC, et al. 2004. Effect of Vitamin D on falls: a meta-analysis. *Journal of the American Medical Association* 291(16):1999-2006.

Garland CF, Garland FC. 1980. Do sunlight and vitamin D reduce the likelihood of colon cancer? *International Journal of Epidemiology* 9(3):227-31.

Grant WB. 2003. Ecologic studies of solar UV-B radiation and cancer mortality rates. *Recent Results in Cancer Research* 164:371-7.

Harris S. 2002. Can vitamin D supplementation in infancy prevent type 1 diabetes? *Nutrition Reviews* 60(4):118-21.

Holick MF, Shao Q, Liu WW, Chen TC. 1992. The vitamin D content of fortified milk and infant formula. *New England Journal of Medicine* 326(18):1178-81.

Holick MF. 2004. Vitamin D: importance in the prevention of cancers, type 1 diabetes, heart disease, and osteoporosis. *American Journal of Clinical Nutrition* 79(5):890.

Holick, Michael, MD, PhD. 2004. Interview with the authors. Oct. 17.

Jiang F, Bao J, Li P, Nicosia SV, Bai W. 2004. Induction of ovarian cancer cell apoptosis by 1,25-dihydroxyvitamin D3 through the down regulation of telomerase. *Journal of Biological Chemistry* Oct 12.

Krishnan AV, Peehl DM, Feldman D. 2003. The role of vitamin D in prostate cancer. *Recent Results Cancer Research* 164:205-21.

Li YC, Qiao G, Uskokovic M, Xiang W, et al. 2004.Vitamin D: a negative endocrine regulator of the renin-angiotensin system and blood pressure. *Journal of Steroid Biochemistry and Molecular Biology* 89-90(1-5):387-92.

Mawer EB, Davies M. 2001. Vitamin D nutrition and bone disease in adults. *Reviews in Endocrine Metabolic Disorders* 2(2):153-64.

National Health and Nutrition Examination Survey. John EM, Schwartz GG, Dreon DM, Koo J. 1999. Vitamin D and breast cancer risk: the NHANES I Epidemiologic follow-up study, 1971-1975 to 1992. *Cancer Epidemiology, Biomarkers and Prevention* 8(5):399-406.

Vieth R. 1999. Vitamin D supplementation, 25-hydroxyvitamin D concentrations, and safety. *American Journal of Clinical Nutrition* 69(5):842-56.

Vieth R. 2004. Why the optimal requirement for Vitamin D3 is probably much higher than what is officially recommended for adults. *Journal of Steroid Biochemistry and Molecular Biology* 89-90(1-5):575-9.

Whitmore SE. 1996. Vitamin D deficiency in homebound elderly persons. *Journal of the American Medical Association* 275(11):838-9.

William B. Grant, PhD. 2004. The role of ultraviolet-B (UVB) radiation (290-315 nm) and vitamin D in reducing the risk of cancer. Submitted for publication, 3/9/2004.

Chapter 25

Ames BN. 2001. DNA damage from micronutrient deficiencies is likely to be a major cause of cancer. *Mutation Research* 475:7-20.

Blount BC, Mack MM, Wehr CM, et al. 1997. Folate deficiency causes uracil misincorporation into human DNA and chromosome breakage: implications for cancer and neuronal damage. *Proceedings of the National Academy of Sciences of the United States of America* 94(7):3290-3295.

Fuchs CS, Willett WC, Colditz GA, et al. 2002. The influence of folate and multivitamin use on the familial risk of colon cancer in women. *Cancer Epidemiology, Biomarkers and Prevention* 11(3):227-34.

Malinow MR, Duell PB, Hess DL, et al. 1998. Reduction of plasma homocyst(e)ine levels by breakfast cereal fortified with folic acid in patients with coronary heart disease. *New England Journal of Medicine* 338(15):1009-15.

Malinow MR, Duell PB, Irvin-Jones A, et al. 2000. Increased plasma homocyst(e)ine after withdrawal of ready-to-eat breakfast cereal from the diet: prevention by breakfast cereal providing 200 microg folic acid. *Journal of the American College of Nutrition* 19(4):452-7.

McFarlane SI, Muniyappa R, Shin JJ, et al. 2004. Osteoporosis and cardiovascular disease: brittle bones and boned arteries, is there a link? *Endocrine* 23(1):1-10.

McLean RR, Jacques PF, Selhub J, et al. 2004. Homocysteine as a predictive factor for hip fracture in older persons. *New England Journal of Medicine* 350(20):2042-9.

Oakley, Godfrey Jr., MD, MPH. 2004.Interview with the authors. Oct. 26.

Russell S. 2004. Folate may curb heart attacks, strokes; B vitamin is added to flour to reduce risk of birth defects. *San Francisco Chronicle*, March 6, 2004.

Taylor MJ, Carney S, Geddes J, et al. 2003. Folate for depressive disorders. *Cochrane Database of Systematic Reviews* (2):CD003390.

Wald DS, Law M, Morris JK. 2004. The dose-response relation between serum homocysteine and cardiovascular disease: implications for treatment and screening. *European Journal of Cardiovascular Prevention and Rehabilitation* 11(3):250-3.

Zhang SM, Willett WC, Selhub J, et al. 2003. Plasma folate, vitamin B6, vitamin B12, homocysteine, and risk of breast cancer. *Journal of the National Cancer Institute* 95(5):373-80.

Chapter 26

Fahey JW, Zhang Y, Talalay P. 1997. Broccoli sprouts: an exceptionally rich source of inducers of enzymes that protect against chemical carcinogens. *Proceedings of the National Academy of the Sciences of the U.S.A.* 94(19):10367-72.

Jenkins DJ, Kendall CW, Marchie A, et al. 2003. Effects of a dietary portfolio of cholesterol-lowering foods vs lovastatin on serum lipids and C-reactive protein. *Journal of the American Medical Association* 290(4):502-10.

Liu RH. 2003. Health benefits of fruit and vegetables are from additive and synergistic combinations of phytochemicals. *American Journal of Clinical Nutrition* 78(3 Suppl):517S-520S.

Mann NJ. 2004. Paleolithic nutrition: what can we learn from the past? *Asia Pacific Journal of Clinical Nutrition* 13(Suppl):S17.

Margen S. and the editors of the UC Berkeley Wellness Letter. 2002. Wellness Foods A-Z: An indispensable guide for health-conscious food lovers. *Health Letter Associates.*

O'Keefe JH Jr, Cordain L. 2004. Cardiovascular disease resulting from a diet and lifestyle at odds with our Paleolithic genome: how to become a 21st-century hunter-gatherer. *Mayo Clinics Proceedings* 79(1):101-8.

Paolisso G, Tagliamonte MR, Rizzo MR, et al. 1998. Oxidative stress and advancing age: results in healthy centenarians. *Journal of the American Geriatric Society* 46(7):833-8.

De Mejia EG, Castano-Tostado E, Loarca-Pina G. 1999. Antimutagenic effects of natural phenolic compounds in beans. *Mutation Research* 441(1):1-9.

Purba MB, Kouris-Blazos A, Wattanapenpaiboon N, et al. 2001. Skin wrinkling: can food make a difference? *Journal of the American College of Nutrition* 20(1):71-80.

Riedel WJ, Jorissen BL. 1998. Nutrients, age and cognitive function. *Current Opinions in Clinical Nutrition and Metabolic Care* 1(6):579-85.

Snowdon, DA, Phillips RL. 1985. Does a vegetarian diet reduce the occurrence of diabetes? *American Journal of Public Health* 75:507-512.

Steinmetz KA, Kushi LH, Bostick RM, et al. 1994. Vegetables, fruit, and colon cancer in the Iowa Women's Health Study. *American Journal of Epidemiology* 139(1):1-15.

Willett W. 2003. Lessons from dietary studies in Adventists and questions for the future. *American Journal of Clinical Nutrition* 78(3 Suppl):539S-543S.

Chapter 27

Cho E, Seddon JM, Rosner B, et al. 2004. Prospective study of intake of fruits, vegetables, vitamins, and carotenoids and risk of age-related maculopathy. *Archives of Ophthalmology* 122(6):883-92.

Commenges D, Scotet V, Renaud S, et al. 2000. Intake of flavonoids and risk of dementia. *European Journal of Epidemiology* 16(4):357-63.

Eaton SB, Eaton SB 3rd. 2000. Paleolithic vs. modern diets—selected pathophysiological implications. *European Journal of Nutrition* 39(2):67-70.

Goyarzu P, Malin DH, Lau FC, et al. 2004. Blueberry supplemented diet: effects on object recognition memory and nuclear factor-kappa B levels in aged rats. *Nutritional Neuroscience* 7(2):75-83.

Joseph JA, Denisova NA, Arendash G, et al. 2003. Blueberry supplementation enhances signaling and prevents behavioral deficits in an Alzheimer disease model. *Nutritional Neuroscience* 6(3):153-62.

Levine SR, Coull BM. 2002. Potassium depletion as a risk factor for stroke: will a banana a day keep your stroke away? *Neurology* 59(3):302-3.

Singh RB, Rastogi SS, Singh NK, et al. 1993. Can guava fruit intake decrease blood pressure and blood lipids? *Journal of Human Hypertension* 7(1):33-8.

Strandhagen E, Hansson PO, Bosaeus I, et al. 2000. High fruit intake may reduce mortality among middle-aged and elderly men. The Study of Men Born in 1913. *European Journal of Clinical Nutrition* 54(4):337-41.

Chapter 28

Anderson JW. 2003. Whole grains protect against atherosclerotic cardiovascular disease. *The Proceedings of the Nutrition Society* 62(1):135-42.

Fung TT, Hu FB, Pereira MA, et al. 2002. Whole-grain intake and the risk of type 2 diabetes: a prospective study in men. *American Journal of Clinical Nutrition.* 76(3):535-40.

Grocery Manufacturers of America. 2004. Grocery Manufacturers of America Comments to the USDA Dietary Guidelines Advisory Committee. www.gmabrands.com/publicpolicy/docs/comment.cfm? DocID=1317

Jacobs DR Jr, Marquart L, Slavin J, et al. 1998. Whole-grain intake and cancer: an expanded review and meta-analysis. *Nutrition and Cancer* 30(2):85-96.

Marlett JA, McBurney MI, Slavin JL; American Dietetic Association. 2002. Position of the American Dietetic Association: health implications of dietary fiber. *Journal of the American Dietetic Association* 102(7):993-1000.

Marquart L, Wiemer KL, Jones JM, et al. 2003. Whole grains health claims in the USA and other efforts to increase whole-grain consumption. *The Proceedings of the Nutritional Society* 62(1):151-60.

Ness, C. 2005. New diet rules rely on common sense; Federal Guidelines emphasize weight, call for more exercise. *San Francisco Chronicle* January 13, 2005.

Slavin J. 2003. Why whole grains are protective: biological mechanisms. *The Proceedings of the Nutritional Society* 62(1):129-34.

Willett W. 2001. *Eat, Drink, and Be Healthy: the Harvard Medical School guide to healthy eating.* Simon & Schuster Source.

Chapter 29

Ajani UA, Ford ES, Mokdad AH. 2004. Dietary fiber and C-reactive protein: findings from national health and nutrition examination survey data. *Journal of Nutrition* 134(5):1181-5.

Aldoori WH, Giovannucci EL, Rockett HR, et al. 1998. A prospective study of dietary fiber types and symptomatic diverticular disease in men. *Journal of Nutrition* 128:714-9.

Bazzano LA, He J, Ogden LG, et al. 2003. Dietary fiber intake and reduced risk of coronary heart disease in US men and women: the National Health and Nutrition Examination Survey I Epidemiologic Follow-up Study. *Archives of Internal Medicine* 163(16):1897-904.

Brown L, Rosner B, Willett WW, et al. 1999. Cholesterol-lowering effects of dietary fiber: a meta-analysis. *American Journal of Clinical Nutrition* 69(1):30-42.

Davy BM, Davy KP, Ho RC, et al. 2002. High-fiber oat cereal compared with wheat cereal consumption favorably alters LDL-cholesterol subclass and particle numbers in middle-aged and older men. *American Journal of Clinical Nutrition* 76(2):351-8.

Fuchs CS, Giovannucci EL, Colditz GA, et al. 1999. Dietary fiber and the risk of colorectal cancer and adenoma in women. *New England Journal of Medicine* 340(3):169-76.

He J, Streiffer RH, Muntner P, et al. 2004. Effect of dietary fiber intake on blood pressure: a randomized, double-blind, placebo-controlled trial. *Journal of Hypertension* 22(1):73-80.

Jimenez-Escrig A, Rincon M, Pulido R, Saura-Calixto F. 2001. Guava fruit (Psidium guajava L.) as a new source of antioxidant dietary fiber. *Journal of Agricultural and Food Chemistry* 49(11):5489-93.

Lupton JR, Turner ND. 2003. Dietary fiber and coronary disease: does the evidence support an association? *Current Atherosclerosis Reports* 5(6):500-5.

Pereira MA, Ludwig DS. 2001. Dietary fiber and body-weight regulation. Observations and mechanisms. *Pediatric Clinics of North America* 48(4):969-80.

Pereira MA, O'Reilly E, Augustsson K, et al. 2004. Dietary fiber and risk of coronary heart disease: a pooled analysis of cohort studies. *Archives of Internal Medicine* 164(4):370-6.

Rimm EB, Ascherio A, Giovannucci E, et al. 1996. Vegetable, fruit, and cereal fiber intake and risk of coronary heart disease among men. *Journal of the American Medical Association* 275:447-51.

Slattery ML, Curtin KP, Edwards SL, et al. 2004. Plant foods, fiber, and rectal cancer. *American Journal of Clinical Nutrition* 79(2):274-81.

Slavin, Joanne, PhD, RD. 2004. Interview with the authors. Nov. 4.

Chapter 30

Anderson C, Heike K, Colquhoun D. 2003. Recommended fish intake is potentially dangerous due to high methylmercury content of certain fish. *Asia Pacific Journal of Clinical Nutrition* 12 Suppl:S67.

Augustsson K, Michaud DS, Rimm EB, et al. 2003. A prospective study of intake of fish and marine fatty acids and prostate cancer. *Cancer Epidemiology, Biomarkers and Prevention* 12(1):64-7.

Bosch X. 1998. Fish consumption and depression. *Lancet* 352(9121):71-2.

Cleland LG, James MJ, Proudman SM. 2003. The role of fish oils in the treatment of rheumatoid arthritis. *Drugs* 63(9):845-53.

De Deckere EA. 1999. Possible beneficial effect of fish and fish n-3 polyunsaturated fatty acids in breast and colorectal cancer. *European Journal of Cancer Prevention* 8(3):213-21.

Fernandez E, Chatenoud L, La Vecchia C, et al. 1999. Fish consumption and cancer risk. *American Journal of Clinical Nutrition* 70(1):85-90.

Geleijnse JM, Giltay EJ, Grobbee DE, et al. 2002. Blood pressure response to fish oil supplementation: metaregression analysis of randomized trials. *Journal of Hypertens*ion 20(8):1493-9.

Hightower, Jane, MD. 2004. Interview with the authors. Nov. 4.

Morris MC, Evans DA, Bienias JL, et al. 2003. Consumption of fish and n-3 fatty acids and risk of incident Alzheimer disease. *Archives of Neurology* 60(7):940-6.

Moszczynski P. 1997. Mercury compounds and the immune system: a review. *International Journal of Occupational Medicine and Environmental Health* 10(3):247-58.

Nkondjock A, Receveur O. 2003. Fish-seafood consumption, obesity, and risk of type 2 diabetes: an ecological study. *Diabetes and Metabolism* 29(6):635-42.

O'Keefe JH Jr, Harris WS. 2000. From Inuit to implementation: omega-3 fatty acids come of age. *Mayo Clinic Proceedings* 75(6):607-14.

Rylander L, Hagmar L. 1995. Mortality and cancer incidence among women with a high consumption of fatty fish contaminated with persistent organochlorine compounds. *Scandinavian Journal of Work and Environmental Health* 21(6):419-26.

Terry P, Wolk A, Vainio H, et al. 2002. Fatty fish consumption lowers the risk of endometrial cancer: a nationwide case-control study in Sweden. *Cancer Epidemiology, Biomarkers and Prevention* 11(1):143-5.

Whelton SP, He J, Whelton PK et al. 2004. Meta-analysis of observational studies on fish intake and coronary heart disease. *American Journal of Cardiology* 93(9):1119-23.

Yoshizawa K, Rimm EB, Morris JS, et al. 2002. Mercury and the risk of coronary heart disease in men. *New England Journal of Medicine* 347(22):1755-60.

Chapter 31

Arvanitakis Z, Wilson RS, Bienias JL, et al. 2004. Diabetes mellitus and risk of Alzheimer disease and decline in cognitive function. *Archives of Neurology* 61(5):661-6.

Dowd SB, Davidhizar R. 2003. Can mental and physical activities such as chess and gardening help in the prevention and treatment of Alzheimer's? Healthy aging through stimulation of the mind. *The Journal of Practical Nursing* 53(3):11-3.

Fratiglioni L, Paillard-Borg S, Winblad B. 2004. An active and socially integrated lifestyle in late life might protect against dementia. *Lancet. Neurology* 3(6):343-53.

Grossman H. 2003. Does diabetes protect or provoke Alzheimer's disease? Insights into the pathobiology and future treatment of Alzheimer's disease. *CNS Spectrums* 8(11):815-23.

Gustafson D, Rothenberg E, Blennow K, et al. 2003. An 18-year follow-up of overweight and risk of Alzheimer disease. *Archives of Internal Medicine* 163(13):1524-8.

Hebert LE, Scherr PA, Bienias JL, et al. 2003. Alzheimer disease in the US population: prevalence estimates using the 2000 census. *Archives of Neurology* 60(8):1119-22.

Honig LS, Tang MX, Albert S, et al. 2003. Stroke and the risk of Alzheimer disease. *Archives of Neurology* 60(12):1707-12.

Malaguarnera M, Ferri R, Bella R, et al. 2004. Homocysteine, vitamin B12 and folate in vascular dementia and in Alzheimer disease. *Clinical Chemistry and Laboratory Medicine* 42(9):1032-5.

Miller LJ, Chacko R. 2004. The role of cholesterol and statins in Alzheimer's disease. *Annals of Pharmacotherapy* 38(1):91-8.

Morris MC, Evans DA, Bienias JL, et al. 2003. Consumption of fish and n-3 fatty acids and risk of incident Alzheimer disease. *Archives of Neurology* 60(7):940-6.

Seshadri S, Beiser A, Selhub J, et al. 2002. Plasma homocysteine as a risk factor for dementia and Alzheimer's disease. *New England Journal of Medicine* 346(7):476-83.

Skoog I, Gustafson D. 2003. Hypertension, hypertension-clustering factors and Alzheimer's disease. *Neurological Research* 25(6):675-80.

Small, Gary, MD. 2004. Interview with the authors. November 1.

Szekely CA, Thorne JE, Zandi PP, et al. 2004. Nonsteroidal anti-inflammatory drugs for the prevention of Alzheimer's disease: a systematic review. *Neuroepidemiology* 23(4):159-69.

Weuve J, Kang JH, Manson JE, et al. 2004. Physical activity, including walking, and cognitive function in older women. *Journal of the American Medical Association* 292(12):1454-61.

Zandi PP, Anthony JC, Khachaturian AS, et al. 2004. Reduced risk of Alzheimer disease in users of antioxidant vitamin supplements: the Cache County Study. *Archives of Neurology* 61(1):82-8.

2004. Study: distress-prone people more likely to develop Alzheimer's disease. *FDA Consumer* 38(1):8.

Chapter 32

Di Castelnuovo A, Rotondo S, Iacoviello L, et al. 2002. Meta-analysis of wine and beer consumption in relation to vascular risk. *Circulation* 105(24):2836-44.

Klatsky AL, Friedman GD, Armstrong MA, Kipp H. 2003. Wine, liquor, beer, and mortality. *American Journal of Epidemiology* 158(6):585-95.

Klatsky AL. 1998. Alcohol and cardiovascular diseases: a historical overview. *Novartis Foundation Symposium* 216:2-12

Klatsky AL. 1999. Moderate drinking and reduced risk of heart disease. *Alcohol Research and Health* 23(1):15-23.

Klatsky AL. 2004. Alcohol-Associated Hypertension: When One Drinks Makes a Difference. *Hypertension* Oct 18

Klatsky AL. J 2003. Alcohol and cardiovascular disease—more than one paradox to consider. Alcohol and hypertension: does it matter? Yes. *Cardiovascular Risk* 10(1):21-4.

Klatsky, Arthur, MD. 2004. Interview with the authors. November 5.

Renaud S, de Lorgeril M. 1992. Wine, alcohol, platelets, and the French paradox for coronary heart disease. *Lancet* 339(8808):1523-6.

Ruitenberg A, van Swieten JC, Witteman JC, et al. 2002. Alcohol consumption and risk of dementia: the Rotterdam Study. *Lancet* 359(9303):281-6.

Stampfer MJ, Kang JH, Chen J, et al. 2005. Effects of moderate alcohol consumption on cognitive function in women. *New England Journal of Medicine* 352(3):245-53.

Truelsen T, Gronbaek M, Schnohr P, Boysen G. 1998. Intake of beer, wine, and spirits and risk of stroke : the copenhagen city heart study. *Stroke* 29(12):2467-72.

Van de Wiel A. 2002. Nutrition and health—favorable effect of wine and wine flavonoids on cardiovascular diseases. *Ned Tijdschr Geneeskd* 146(51):2466-9.

Chapter 33

Bener A, Alwash R, Gaber T, Lovasz G. 2003. Obesity and low back pain. *Collegium Antropologicum* 27(1):95-104.

Carpenter DM, Nelson BW. 1999. Low back strengthening for the prevention and treatment of low back pain. *Medicine and Science in Sports and Exercise* 31(1):18-24.

Goldberg MS, Scott SC, Mayo NE. 2000. A review of the association between cigarette smoking and the development of nonspecific back pain and related outcomes. *Spine* 25(8):995-1014.

Lahad A, Malter AD, Berg AO, Deyo RA. 1994. The effectiveness of four interventions for the prevention of low back pain. *Journal of the American Medical Association* 272(16):1286-91.

Sculco AD, Paup DC, Fernhall B, Sculco MJ. 2001. Effects of aerobic exercise on low back pain patients in treatment. *Spine Journal* 1(2):95-101.

Van Poppel MN, Hooftman WE, Koes BW. 2004. An update of a systematic review of controlled clinical trials on the primary prevention of back pain at the workplace. *Occupational Medicine (London)* 54(5):345-52.

Winett RA, Carpinelli RN. 2001. Potential health-related benefits of resistance training. *Preventitive Medicine* 33(5):503-13.

Chapter 34
American Dietetic Association; Dietitians of Canada. 2003. Position of the American Dietetic Association and Dietitians of Canada: vegetarian diets. *Canadian Journal of Dietetic Practice and Research* 2003 64(2):62-81.

Appleby PN, Thorogood M, Mann JI, et al. 1999. The Oxford Vegetarian Study: an overview. *American Journal of Clinical Nutrition* 70(3 Suppl):525S-531S.

Fraser GE. 1999. Associations between diet and cancer, ischemic heart disease, and all-cause mortality in non-Hispanic white California Seventh-day Adventists. *American Journal of Clinical Nutrition* 70(3 Suppl):532S-538S.

Giem P, Beeson WL, Fraser GE. 1993. The incidence of dementia and intake of animal products: preliminary findings from the Adventist Health Study. *Neuroepidemiology* 12(1):28-36.

Glade MJ. 1997. Food, Nutrition and the Prevention of Cancer: A Global Perspective. *World Cancer Research Fund/the American Institute for Cancer Research.*

Itoh R, Nishiyama N, Suyama Y. 1998. Dietary protein intake and urinary excretion of calcium: a cross-sectional study in a healthy Japanese population. *American Journal of Clinical Nutrition* 67(3):438-44.

Ross GW, Petrovitch H, White LR, et al. 1999. Characterization of risk factors for vascular dementia: the Honolulu-Asia Aging Study. *Neurology* 53(2):337-43.

Chapter 35
Bassett DR, Schneider PL, Huntington GE. 2004. Physical activity in an Old Order Amish community. *Medicine and Science in Sports and Exercise* 36(1):79-85.

Farrell SW, Braun L, Barlow CE, Cheng YJ, et al. 2002. The relation of body mass index, cardiorespiratory fitness, and all-cause mortality in women. *Obesity Research* 10(6):417-23.

Katzel LI, Bleecker ER, Colman EG, et al. 1995. Effects of weight loss vs. aerobic exercise training on risk factors for coronary disease in healthy, obese, middle-aged and older men. *Journal of the American Medical Association* 274:1915-21.

Kelner and Helmuth. 2003. Obesity - What Is To Be Done? *Science* 299: 845.

Killingsworth RE. 2003. Health promoting community design: a new paradigm to promote healthy and active communities. *American Journal of Health Promotion* 17(3):169-70, ii.

Klem ML, Wing RR, McGuire MT, et al. 1997. A descriptive study of individuals successful at long-term maintenance of substantial weight loss. *American Journal of Clinical Nutrition* 66:239-46.

Kolotkin RL, Crosby RD, Williams GR, et al. 2001. The relationship between health-related quality of life and weight loss. *Obesity Research* 9(9):564-71.

Rolls BJ, Bell EA, Thorwart ML. 1999. Water incorporated into a food but not served with a food decreases energy intake in lean women. *American Journal of Clinical Nutrition* 70(4):448-55.

Rolls, Barbara, PhD. 2004. Interview with the authors. November 11.

Sorensen TI. 2003. Weight loss causes increased mortality: pros. *Obesity Review* 4(1):3-7.

Utter AC, Nieman DC, Shannonhouse EM, et al. 1998. Influence of diet and/or exercise on body composition and cardiorespiratory fitness in obese women. *International Journal of Sport Nutrition* 8(3):213-22.

Chapter 36

Kral T, Roe L, Rolls B. 2003. The Combined Effect of Energy Density and Portion Size on Food and Energy Intake in Women. *University of Pennsylvania Laboratory for the Study of Human Ingestive Behaviors. Presented at the 2003 annual meeting of the North American Association for the Study of Obesity.*

Kral T, Meengs JS, Wall DE. 2003. Effect on Food Intake of Increasing the Portion Size of All Foods Over Two Consecutive Days. *University of Pennsylvania Laboratory for the Study of Human Ingestive Behaviors. Presented at the 2003 Experimental Biology Conference.*

Nielsen SJ, Popkin BM. 2004. Changes in beverage intake between 1977 and 2001. *American Journal Preventitive Medicine* 27(3):205-10.

Nielsen SJ, Popkin BM. Patterns and trends in food portion sizes, 1977-1998. 2003. *Journal of the American Medical Association* 289(4):450-3.

Rolls BJ, Ello-Martin JA, Tohill BC. 2004. What can intervention studies tell us about the relationship between fruit and vegetable consumption and weight management? *Nutrition Reviews* 62(1):1-17.

Rolls BJ, Roe LS, Meengs JS, et al. 2004. Increasing the portion size of a sandwich increases energy intake. *Journal of the American Dietetic Association* 104(3):367-72.

Rolls BJ, Roe LS, Meengs JS. 2004. Salad and satiety: energy density and portion size of a first-course salad affect energy intake at lunch. *Journal of the American Dietetic Association* 104(10):1570-6.

Rolls, Barbara, PhD. 2004. Interview with the authors. November 11.

Chapter 37

Alvarez GG, Ayas NT. 2004. The impact of daily sleep duration on health: a review of the literature. *Progress in Cardiovascular Nursing* 19(2):56-9.

Cohen S, Doyle WJ, Skoner DP, et al. 1997. Social ties and susceptibility to the common cold. *Journal of the American Medical Association* 277(24):1940-4.

Kushida, Clete, MD, PhD. 2004. Interview with the authors. Nov. 11.

Moldofsky H. 1995. Sleep and the immune system. *International Journal of Immunopharmacology* 17(8):649-54.

Parish JM, Somers VK. 2004. Obstructive sleep apnea and cardiovascular disease. *Mayo Clinic Proceedings* 79(8):1036-46.

Pilcher JJ, Huffcutt AI. 1996. Effects of sleep deprivation on performance: a meta-analysis. *Sleep* 19(4):318-26.

Ribeiro S, Gervasoni D, Soares ES, et al. 2004. Long-Lasting Novelty-Induced Neuronal Reverberation during Slow-Wave Sleep in Multiple Forebrain Areas. *PLoS Biology.* 2(1):E24. Epub 2004 Jan 20.

Urponen H, Vuori I, Hasan J, Partinen M. 1988. Self-evaluations of factors promoting and disturbing sleep: an epidemiological survey in Finland. *Social Science and Medicine* 26(4):443-50.

Wagner U, Gais S, Haider H, Verleger R, et al. 2004. Sleep inspires insight. *Nature* 427(6972):352-5.

Young T, Peppard PE, Gottlieb DJ. 2002. Epidemiology of obstructive sleep apnea: a population health perspective. *American Journal of Respiratory and Critical Care Medicine* 165(9):1217-39.

Youngstedt SD, O'Connor PJ, Dishman RK. 1997. The effects of acute exercise on sleep: a quantitative synthesis. *Sleep* 20(3):203-14.

Chapter 38

Bryant S, Rakowski W. 1992. Predictors of mortality among elderly African Americans. *Research on Aging* 14:50-67.

Ellison CG, Hummer RA, Cormier S, et al. 2000. Religious involvement and mortality risk among African American adults. *Research on Aging* 22:630-667.

Griffith D, Baker EA, Strayhorn S, et al. 2004. Churches as structures of social support for healthier eating. *School of Public Health, Saint Louis University. Presentation at the annual meeting of the American Public Health Association, Nov. 9, 2004.*

Hummer RA, Rogers RG, Nam CB, et al. 1999. Religious involvement and U.S. adult mortality. *Demography* 36(2):273-85.

Hummer, Robert, PhD. 2004. Interview with the authors. November 8.

Koenig H.G., Ford S., George L.K., et al. 1993. Religion and anxiety disorder: An examination and comparison of associations in young, middle-aged, and elderly adults. *Journal of Anxiety Disorders* 7:321-342.

Koenig H.G., Hays J.C., George L.K et al. 1997. Modeling the cross-sectional relationships between religion, physical health, social support, and depressive symptoms. *American Journal of Geriatric Psychiatry* 5:131-143.

Lutgendorf SK, Russell D, Ullrich P, et al. 2004. Religious participation, interleukin-6, and mortality in older adults. *Health Psychology* 23(5):465-75.

Sloan RP, Bagiella E. 2002. Claims about religious involvement and health outcomes. *Annals of Behavioral Medicine* 24(1):14-21. (NIB).

Strawbridge WJ, Cohen RD, Shema SJ, et al. 1997. Frequent attendance at religious services and mortality over 28 years. *American Journal of Public Health* 87(6):957-61.

Strawbridge WJ, Cohen RD, Shema SJ. 2000. Comparative strength of association between religious attendance and survival. *International Journal of Psychiatry Medicine* 30(4):299-308.

Chapter 39

Bortz, Walter M., MD. 2004. Interview with the authors. November 9.

Gerwood JB. 1998. The legacy of Viktor Frankl: an appreciation upon his death. *Psychological Reports* 82(2):673-4.

Hasegawa A, Fujiwara Y, Hoshi T, Shinkai S. 2003. Regional differences in *ikigai* (reason(s) for living) in elderly people—relationship between *ikigai* and family structure, physiological situation and functional capacity. *Nippon Ronen Igakkai Zasshi* 40(4):390-6.

Krause N. 2004. Stressors arising in highly valued roles, meaning in life, and the physical health status of older adults. *Journal of Gerontology, Series B, Psychological Sciences and Social Sciences* 59(5):S287-97.

Seki N. 2001. Relationships between walking hours, sleeping hours, meaningfulness of life (*ikigai*) and mortality in the elderly: prospective cohort study. *Nippon Eiseigaku Zasshi* 56(2):535-40.

Takkinen S, Ruoppila I. 2001. Meaning in life in three samples of elderly persons with high cognitive functioning. *International Journal of Aging and Human Development* 53(1):51-73.

Ventegodt S, Andersen NJ, Merrick J. 2003. Quality of life philosophy V. Seizing the meaning of life and becoming well again. *Scientific World Journal* 3:1210-29.

Yoshida K. 1994. Evaluation of a revised *"Ikigai"* scale and the relationship between motivation for achievement of a purpose and mental health in senior high school students. *Nippon Koshu Eisei Zasshi* 41(12):1162-

8.

Chapter 40

Brennemann J. 1932. The Infant Ward. *American Journal of Diseases of Children* 43. (577).

Delaney J.P., Leong K.S., Watkins A., & Brodie D. 2002. The short-term effects of myofascial trigger point massage therapy on cardiac autonomic tone in healthy subjects. *Journal of Advanced Nursing* 37:364-71.

Diego M.A., Hernandez-Reif M., Field T., Friedman L. & Shaw K. 2001. HIV adolescents show improved immune function following massage therapy. *International Journal of Neuroscience* 106:35-45.

Field, Tiffany, PhD. 2004. Interview with the authors. August 16.

Hernandez-Reif M., Ironson G., Field T., Katz G., Diego M., Weiss S., Fletcher M., Schanberg S. & Kuhn C. (In Review). Breast cancer patients have improved immune functions following massage therapy.

Ironson G., Field T., Scafidi F., Hashimoto M., Kumar M., Kumar A., Price A., Goncalves A., Burman I., Tetenman C., Patarca R., & Fletcher M. A. 1996. Massage therapy is associated with enhancement of the immune system's cytotoxic capacity. *International Journal of Neuroscience* 84:205-217.

Jourard S.M. 1966. An exploratory study of body-accessibility. *British Journal of Social and Clinical Psychology* 2(4):69-75.

Ornish, Dean, MD. 2004. Interview with the authors. August 5.

Verhoef M.J., & Page S.A. 1998. Physicians' perspectives on massage therapy. *Canadian Family Physician* 44.

Chapter 41

Bjelland I, Tell GS, Vollset SE, et al. 2003. Folate, vitamin B12, homocysteine, and the MTHFR 677C->T polymorphism in anxiety and depression: the Hordaland Homocysteine Study. *Archives of General Psychiatry* 60(6):618-26.

Koehler KM, Pareo-Tubbeh SL, Romero LJ, et al. 1997. Folate nutrition and older adults: challenges and opportunities. *Journal of the American Dietetic Association* 97(2):167-73.

McCully KS. 1969. Vascular pathology of homocysteinemia: implications for the pathogenesis of arteriosclerosis. *American Journal of Pathology* 56(1):111-28.

Morris MS. 2003. Homocysteine and Alzheimer's disease. *Lancet. Neurology* 2(7):425-8.

Selhub J, Jacques PF, Bostom AG, et al. 1995. Association between plasma homocysteine concentrations and extracranial carotid-artery stenosis. *New England Journal of Medicine* 332(5):286-91.

Seshadri S, Beiser A, Selhub J, et al. 2002. Plasma homocysteine as a risk factor for dementia and Alzheimer's disease. *New England Journal of Medicine* 346(7):476-83.

van Meurs JB, Dhonukshe-Rutten RA, Pluijm SM, et al. 2004. Homocysteine levels and the risk of osteoporotic fractures. *New England Journal of Medicine* May 13.

Verhoef P, Stampfer MJ, Buring JE, et al. 1996. Homocysteine metabolism and risk of myocardial infarction: relation with vitamins B6, B12, and folate. *American Journal of Epidemiology* 143(9):845-59.

Chapter 42

Abramson, Mark, MD. Interview with the authors. November 18.

Barnes VA, Treiber FA, Johnson MH. 2004. Impact of transcendental meditation on ambulatory blood pressure in African-American adolescents. *American Journal of Hypertension* 17(4):366-9.

Creamer P, Singh BB, Hochberg MC, et al. 2000. Sustained improvement produced by nonpharmacologic intervention in fibromyalgia: results of a pilot study. *Arthritis Care Research* 13(4):198-204.

Davidson RJ, Kabat-Zinn J, Schumacher J, et al. 2003. Alterations in brain and immune function produced by mindfulness meditation. *Psychosomatic Medicine* 65(4):564-70.

Kabat-Zinn J, Lipworth L, Burney R. 1985. The clinical use of mindfulness meditation for the self-regulation of chronic pain. *Journal of Behavioral Medicine* 8(2):163-90.

Kabat-Zinn J, Wheeler E, Light T, et al. 1998. Influence of a mindfulness meditation-based stress reduction intervention on rates of skin clearing in patients with moderate to severe psoriasis undergoing phototherapy (UVB) and photochemotherapy (PUVA). *Psychosomatic Medicine* 60(5):625-32.

Kaplan KH, Goldenberg DL, Galvin-Nadeau M. 1993. The impact of a meditation-based stress reduction program on fibromyalgia. *General Hospital Psychiatry* 15(5):284-9.

Miller JJ, Fletcher K, Kabat-Zinn J. 1995. Three-year follow-up and clinical implications of a mindfulness meditation-based stress reduction intervention in the treatment of anxiety disorders. *General Hospital Psychiatry* 17(3):192-200.

Reiche EM, Nunes SO. 2004. Morimoto HK. Stress, depression, the immune system, and cancer. *Lancet. Oncology* 5(10):617-25.

Saxe GA, Hebert JR, Carmody JF, et al. 2001. Can diet in conjunction with stress reduction affect the rate of increase in prostate specific antigen after biochemical recurrence of prostate cancer? *The Journal of Urology* 166(6):2202-7.

Sudsuang R, Chentanez V, Veluvan K. 1991. Effect of Buddhist meditation on serum cortisol and total protein levels, blood pressure, pulse rate, lung volume and reaction time. *Physiology and Behavior* 50(3):543-8.

Sun TF, Kuo CC, Chiu NM. 2002. Mindfulness meditation in the control of severe headache. *Chang Gung Medical Journal* 25(8):538-41.

Vyas R, Dikshit N. 2002. Effect of meditation on respiratory system, cardiovascular system and lipid profile. *Indian Journal of Physiology and Pharmacology* 46(4):487-91.

Chapter 43

Bedscapes.com. Bedscapes healing environments: research results. www.bedscapes.com/research.htm.

Fredrickson LM, Anderson DM. 1999. A qualitative exploration of the wilderness experience as a source of spiritual inspiration. *Journal of Environmental Psychology* 19(1):21-39.

Hartig T, Evans G, Jamner L, et al. 2003. Tracking restoration in natural and urban field settings. *Journal of Environmental Psychology* June. 109-123.

Kaplan S. 1995. The restorative benefits of nature: Toward an integrative framework. *Journal of Environmental Psychology* September. 169-182.

Parsons R, Tassinary L, Ulrich R, et al. 1998. The view from the road: Implications for stress recovery and immunization. *Journal of Environmental Psychology* June. 113-140.

Tennessen CM, Cimprich B. 1995. Views to nature: effects on attention. *Journal of Environmental Psychology* 5(1):77-85.

Ulrich RS, Simons RF, Losito BD et al. 1991. Stress Recovery during exposure to natural and urban environments. *Journal of Environmental Psychology* 11.

Ulrich RS. 1984. View from a window may influence recovery from surgery. *Science* 224:420-421.

Warber S, Irvine K. 2002. Greening healthcare: Practicing as if the natural environment really mattered. *Alternative Therapies* Sept/Oct. 76-83.

Warber, Sara, MD. 2004. Interview with the authors. November 23.

Chapter 44

Fein O. 1995. The influence of social class on health status: American and British research on health inequalities. *Journal of General Internal Medicine* 10(10):577-86.

Redelmeier, D. 2001. Interview on CBC Radio One by Mary Lou Finlay. May 14, 2001.

Kaprio J, Sarna S, Fogelholm M, Koskenvuo M. 1996. Total and occupationally active life expectancies in relation to social class and marital status in men classified as healthy at 20 in Finland. *Journal of Epidemiology and Community Health* 50(6):653-60.

Lantz PM, House JS, Lepkowski JM, et al. 1998. Socioeconomic factors, health behaviors, and mortality: results from a nationally representative prospective study of US adults. *Journal of the American Medical Association* 279(21):1703-8.

Marmot MG, Kogevinas M, Elston MA. 1987. Social/economic status and disease. *Annual Review of Public Health* 8:111-35.

Marmot MG, Smith GD, Stansfeld S, et al. 1991. Health inequalities among British civil servants: the Whitehall II study. *Lancet* 337(8754):1387-93.

Redelmeier DA, Singh SM. 2001. Survival in Academy Award-winning actors and actresses. *Annals of Internal Medicine* 15;134(10):955-62.

Chapter 45

Colligan, R. PhD. 2004. Email correspondence to authors, Nov. 24, 2004.

Giltay EJ, Geleijnse JM, Zitman FG, et al. 2004. Dispositional optimism and all-cause and cardiovascular mortality in a prospective cohort of elderly dutch men and women. *Archives of General Psychiatry* 61(11):1126-35.

Maruta T, Colligan RC, Malinchoc M, Offord KP. 2002. Optimism-pessimism assessed in the 1960s and self-reported health status 30 years later. *Mayo Clinic Proceedings* 77(8):748-53.

Mulkana SS, Hailey BJ. 2001. The role of optimism in health-enhancing behavior. *American Journal of Health Behavior* 25(4):388-95.

Scheier MF, Matthews KA, Owens JF, et al. 1989. Dispositional optimism and recovery from coronary artery bypass surgery: the beneficial effects on physical and psychological well-being. *Journal of Personality and Social Psychology* 57(6):1024-40.

Schofield P, Ball D, Smith JG, et al. 2004. Optimism and survival in lung carcinoma patients. *Cancer* 100(6):1276-82.

Segerstrom SC, Taylor SE, Kemeny ME, Fahey JL. 1998. Optimism is associated with mood, coping, and immune change in response to stress. *Journal of Personality and Social Psychology* 74(6):1646-55.

Seligman ME. 2000. Optimism, pessimism, and mortality. *Mayo Clinic Proceedings* 75(2):133-4.

Sumi K. 1997. Optimism, social support, stress, and physical and psychological well-being in Japanese women. *Psychological Reports* 81(1):299-306.

Chapter 46

Brown MJ, Ferruzzi MG, Nguyen ML, et al. 2004. Carotenoid bioavailability is higher from salads ingested with full-fat than with fat-reduced salad dressings as measured with electrochemical detection. *American Journal of Clinical Nutrition* 80(2):396-403.

Covington MB. 2004. Omega-3 fatty acids. *American Family Physician* 70(1):133-40.

Hu FB, Cho E, Rexrode KM, et al. 2003. Fish and long-chain omega-3 fatty acid intake and risk of coronary heart disease and total mortality in diabetic women. *Circulation* 107(14):1852-7.

Kalmijn S, van Boxtel MP, Ocke M, et al. 2004. Dietary intake of fatty acids and fish in relation to cognitive performance at middle age. *Neurology* 62(2):275-80.

Kris-Etherton PM, Harris WS, Appel LJ. 2002. Fish consumption, fish oil, omega-3 fatty acids, and cardiovascular disease. *Circulation* 106(21):2747-57.

Kris-Etherton PM, Zhao G, Binkoski AE, et al. 2001. The effects of nuts on coronary heart disease risk. *Nutrition Reviews* 59(4):103-11.

Thies F, Garry JM, Yaqoob P, et al. 2003. Association of n-3 polyunsaturated fatty acids with stability of atherosclerotic plaques: a randomised controlled trial. *Lancet* 361(9356):477-85.

Chapter 47

Ascherio A, Rimm EB, Hernan MA, et al. 1998. Intake of potassium, magnesium, calcium, and fiber and risk of stroke among US men. *Circulation* 98(12):1198-1204.

Appel LJ. 2004. Dietary Reference Intakes: Water, Potassium, Sodium, Chloride, and Sulfate. Institute of Medicine. February 2004.

Delgado MC. 2004. Potassium in hypertension. *Current Hypertension Reports* 6(1):31-5.

Food and Nutrition Board, Institute of Medicine. 1997. Calcium. *Dietary Reference Intakes: Calcium, Phosphorus, Magnesium, Vitamin D, and Fluoride*. Washington, D.C.: National Academy Press; 1997:71-145.

Food and Nutrition Board, Institute of Medicine. 2000. Selenium. *Dietary reference intakes for vitamin C, vitamin E, selenium, and carotenoids*. Washington D.C.: National Academy Press; 2000:284-324.

Gums JG. 2004. Magnesium in cardiovascular and other disorders. *American Journal of Health-System Pharmacy* 61(15):1569-76.

Khaw KT, Barrett-Connor E. 1987. Dietary potassium and stroke-associated mortality. A 12-year prospective population study. *New England Journal of Medicine* 316(5):235-40.

New SA, Robins SP, Campbell MK, et al. 2000. Dietary influences on bone mass and bone metabolism: further evidence of a positive link between fruit and vegetable consumption and bone health? *American Journal of Clinical Nutrition* 71(1):142-151.

Rayman MP, Clark LC. Selenium in cancer prevention. In Roussel AM, ed. *Trace elements in man and animals* 10th ed. New York: Plenum Press; 2000:575-580.

Rayman MP. 2000. The importance of selenium to human health. *Lancet* 356(9225):233-41.

Roy M, Kiremidjian-Schumacher L, Wishe HI, et al. 1994. Supplementation with selenium and human immune cell functions. I. Effect on lymphocyte proliferation and interleukin 2 receptor expression. *Biological Trace Element Research* 41(1-2):103-114.

Sebastian A, Harris ST, Ottaway JH, et al. 1994. Improved mineral balance and skeletal metabolism in postmenopausal women treated with potassium bicarbonate. *New England Journal of Medicine* 330: 1776-1781.

Yokota K, Kato M, Lister F, et al. 2004. Clinical efficacy of magnesium supplementation in patients with type 2 diabetes. *Journal of the American College of Nutrition* 23(5):506S-509S.

Chapter 48

Gardner J, Hallam K. 1999. IOM report lit a fuse. Medical errors are not new, but the very public ruckus over them is; that worries providers. *Modern Healthcare* 29(51):2-3, 12.

Health Grades, Inc. 2002. Health Grades Quality Study, Patient Safety in American Hospitals. www.healthgrades.com. Accessed July 2002.

Institute of Medicine. 1999. *To Err is Human: Building a Safer Health System.* Washington D.C.: National Academy Press, 1999.

Levin, Arthur, MPH. 2004. Interview with the authors. July 20.

Starfield B. 2000. Deficiencies in US medical care. *Journal of the American Medical Association* 284(17):2184-5.

Starfield B. 2000. Is US health really the best in the world? *Journal of the American Medical Association* 284(4):483-5.

Chapter 49

Centers for Disease Control. 2004. Carbon monoxide poisoning: what's the problem? http://www.cdc.gov/nceh/airpollution/carbonmonox-ide/cofaq.hrm.

Howland J, Hingson R. 1988. Alcohol as a risk factor for drownings: A review of the literature (1950–1985). *Accident; Analyis and Prevention* 20(1):19–25.

Litovitz TL, Klein-Schwartz W, White S, et al. 2000 Annual Report of the American Association of Poison Control Centers Toxic Exposures Surveillance System. *American Journal of Emergency Medicine* 19(5): 337-396.

Roberts P, Ward M, Baron RL, et al. 2004. Carbon Monoxide Poisonings Resulting from Open Air Exposures to Operating Motorboats—Lake Havasu City, Arizona, 2003. MMWR 2004; 53(15):314-8. Available at http://www.cdc.gov/mmwr/preview/mmwrhtml/mm5315a3.htm

Shults RA, Elder RW, Sleet DA, et al. 2001. Task Force on Community Preventive Services. Reviews of evidence regarding interventions to reduce alcohol-impaired driving. *American Journal of Preventive Medicine* 2(4 Suppl):66–88.

Chapter 50

Corliss R, Lemonick M. 2004. How To Live To Be 100; New research suggests that a long life is no accident. So what are the secrets of the world's centenarians. *Time* August 30.

Fontaine KR, Redden DT, Wang C, Westfall AO, Allison DB. 2003. Years of life lost due to obesity. *Journal of the American Medical Association* 289:187-93.

Fraser GE, Shavlik DJ. 2001. Ten years of life: is it a matter of choice? *Archives of Internal Medicine* 161:1645-52.

Ljungquist B, Berg S, Lanke J, McClearn GE, Pedersen NL. 1998. The effect of genetic factors for longevity: a comparison of identical and fraternal twins in the Swedish Twin Registry. [PMID: 9823748] *Journal of Gerontology. Series A, Biological Sciences and Medical Sciences* 53:441-6.

Perls T, Kunkel LM, Puca AA. 2002. The genetics of exceptional human longevity. *Journal of the American Geriatric Society* 50:359-68.

Perls TT, Wilmoth J, Levenson R, et al. 2002. Life-long sustained mortality advantage of siblings of centenarians. *Proceedings of the National Academy of the Sciences of the U.S.A.* 99(12):8442-7.

Sho H. 2001. History and characteristics of Okinawan longevity food. *Asia Pacific Journal of Clinical Nutrition* 10(2):159-64.

Suzuki M, Wilcox BJ, Wilcox CD. 2001. Implications from and for food cultures for cardiovascular disease: longevity. *Asia Pacific Journal of Clinical Nutrition* 10(2):165-71.

Index

ABOUT THE AUTHORS

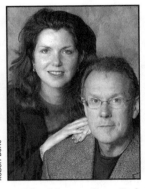

Robert Buric

Suzanne Bohan is an experienced health and science journalist. She serves as a correspondent for the *Sacramento Bee* and worked as a health reporter for ANG Newspapers. She's also contributed to the *San Francisco Chronicle*, *San Jose Mercury News*, and National Public Radio's San Francisco affiliate, KQED. She's won several journalism awards, most recently the 2005 David Perlman Award for Excellence in Medical Journalism. Bohan earned a master's degree in journalism from Stanford University and a bachelor's degree in biology from San Francisco State University.

Glenn Thompson, a graduate of the University of Michigan School of Business, received his law degree from Santa Clara University. He practiced law for two decades while owning and operating radio stations. He's also a devoted student of health and longevity, and has served as a health advocate. Publishing a book about simple ways people can extend their lives has been a goal for more than a decade.

The authors are married and live in Mill Valley, California.